Framing Sexual Dysfunctions and Diseases during Fertility Treatment

Elena Vittoria Longhi

Framing Sexual Dysfunctions and Diseases during Fertility Treatment

A Guide for Healthcare Providers

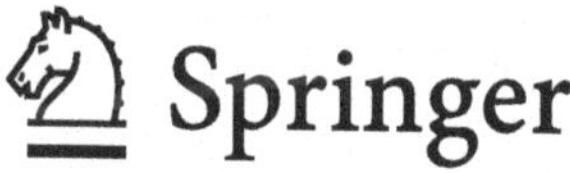

Elena Vittoria Longhi
Sexual Medical Center
San Raffaele Hospital
Milano, Italy

ISBN 978-3-031-76728-9 ISBN 978-3-031-76726-5 (eBook)
https://doi.org/10.1007/978-3-031-76726-5

The original submitted manuscript has been translated into English. The translation was done using artificial intelligence. A subsequent revision was performed by the author(s) to further refine the work and to ensure that the translation is appropriate concerning content and scientific correctness. It may, however, read stylistically different from a conventional translation.

This Springer imprint is published by the registered company Springer Nature Switzerland AG
The registered company address is: Gewerbestrasse 11, 6330 Cham, Switzerland

Foreword 1

The introduction of the contraceptive pill and the consequent prevention of procreation have revolutionized sexuality in Western countries, breaking this centuries-old binomial: sexuality and fertility. With the greater sexual freedom obtained, the age at which we seek to procreate has been pushed back, from the age of 18–22 years in the past to beyond the age of 30 today. According to global statistics, the Italian male seeking offspring is among the oldest in the world: in 2014, he was over 35 years old (ISTAT data).

In the study of the infertile couple, the sexual aspect is rarely evaluated in depth. With current techniques of procreation, the sexual aspect of infertility can be completely ignored, indeed, often it is the couples who do not want to face the problem and want to focus only on fertilization. However, infertility itself can cause sexual disorders. In males, sexuality and fertility are more closely linked than in women. The mechanism of ejaculation, in fact, essential for procreation, requires an orgasm, while a woman can become pregnant even without experiencing any sexual pleasure. The absolute obligation on the part of the male to achieve maximum arousal and an orgasm on command both in diagnostics (semen analysis) and in frequent targeted intercourse often creates a disturbance of pleasure and secondarily of desire. In the most severe cases, it leads to a secondary erectile dysfunction. In literature, there are relatively few authors who deal with this topic, especially in the examination of the sexual causes of infertility.

Every couple has a family history, a personal clinical and emotional experience, as well as the baggage of social relationships. Associated with this are the experiences of the previous relational stories of the individuals and the history of the couple.

With this book, my friend Elena has shown, as usual, a remarkable sensitivity and ability to communicate, offering multiple points of reflection. This guide deals with the topic of fertility in a truly holistic way. It also addresses topics such as the trauma of failure, which can often negatively affect the couple's relationship.

Promea Institute
Turin, Italy

Giorgio Del Noce

Foreword 2

The decline in birth rates and the consequent demographic decrease in Western countries over the last few decades represent an objective fact, potentially responsible for imposing changes to the social, ethnic, and even economic balances of entire societies in different countries. In fact, current estimates from the World Health Organization (WHO) indicate that 72,400,000 people worldwide are involved, that is, 10–15% of couples of reproductive age. The phenomenon is the subject of multidisciplinary studies aimed at identifying its causes, potentially the expression of environmental changes, alterations in lifestyles, sociological and cultural aspects capable of impacting on the dynamics of human reproduction. It should also be considered that, despite the progress of technology and medical science having allowed improvement in the duration and quality of life of men and women, they are still not able to modify a biological clock consolidated throughout the entire evolution of our species. In this context, the reproduction specialist is faced with causal conditions of couple sterility that are difficult to treat and, in many cases, not solvable with medical or surgical therapies, hence the rise in the use of medically assisted reproduction (MAR) techniques as the only and last chance of conception for the infertile couple. This is a path with high costs of a biological, economic, and psychological nature. There is also a risk of decontextualizing the reproductive dynamic from the sexual one, introducing a bias, sometimes of training, to separate drives and elements that nature has established as indissoluble.

This text aims to reunify, in a holistic spirit, two parallel aspects of a single reality: sexuality and reproduction. The psychological difficulties that can negatively impact the sexuality of a couple facing the MAR journey are obvious, but alongside these, there are others, often similar in etiology, and inseparable. Such aspects need to be considered in a single context with the aim of offering infertile couples not only the chance of parenthood but also of satisfying sexuality, in a context burdened by biologically and psychologically unfavorable elements. The topics covered range from comorbidities, to oncology, to lifestyles, and to psychological and relational aspects, potentially impacting on the sexual dynamics of couples who can be included in a medically assisted procreation program. The intention of the editors is to provide a useful tool for daily clinical practice for specialists who are in charge of the infertile couple, shedding new light on related issues that, although correlated, may be misunderstood if the only goal is to have a babe in arms, at any cost, erroneously relegating sexuality to a secondary aspect in the management of the infertile couple.

S.S.D. Pathophysiology of Human Reproduction (MAR) Fabrizio I. Scroppo
San Paolo Hospital, University Center,
Milan, Italy

Foreword 3

In 2023, Human Reproduction Programme (HRP) published a report on the estimated prevalence of infertility worldwide. This document states that about one in six people, or 17.5% of the world's population, is affected by infertility issues. These can lead a person to have difficulty in having a child. Today, thanks to scientific literature, we know the psychological consequences that infertility has on people's lives and the extent of their impact. Research and scientific societies have highlighted this problem, bringing more and more attention to the psychological consequences for individuals and couples.

Even the Ministerial Guidelines are now highlighting the importance of psychological support in this area, but perhaps a step forward should be taken: psychological support may not be enough, and therefore, sexological support may also be needed.

Sexuality has a central aspect in people's lives. First, thanks to contraception, sexuality has become "free" from reproduction, now reproduction has also become "free" from sexuality, thanks to medically assisted reproduction (MAR). However, the impact of infertility has a cost on sexuality, just as a lack of sexuality has a cost on reproductive possibilities. The Nice Guidelines, as we find in the chapter "Principles of Care," draw attention to the fact that couples and individuals must be informed about how both the experience of infertility and MAR techniques affect the sexual life of couples.

In this book, the author addresses the various experiences due to infertility, the characteristics of coping, the importance of preservation in the case of oncological diseases, and places the right attention in observing how fundamental is not only a psychological but also a psychosexual intervention.

The psychosexologist has also in his "toolbox" other tools to accompany the couple in this journey, because as the World Health Organization says: "Reproductive health is a state of complete physical, mental and social well-being and not merely the absence of disease or infirmity, in all matters relating to the reproductive system and its functions and processes. Reproductive health implies that people are able to have a satisfying and safe sexual life and that they have the ability to reproduce and the freedom to decide if, when and how often to do so."

A satisfying sexual life and physical and emotional well-being are the main aspects of people's lives; unfortunately, MAR techniques do not always help in achieving the couple's parenting project, but life goes on and, taking a cue from an aphorism by Aristophanes that says, "The wise man learns many things from his enemies," even from the experience of infertility, many things can be learned. Primarily self-love, then acceptance and the possibility of welcoming a different way of being parents, and finally also the idea of not having children. Acceptance of biological mourning allows us to detach motherhood and fatherhood from genetics and at the same time facilitates the acceptance of gamete donation. Quoting Erich Fromm, "adult love is the ability to give without constraints and demands," that is, to give as a gift, therefore to love also the gift of donation. In other words, the doors are open to building a new story, a story that will concern the future, that is, a child who will continue our love.

After all, even in the successes of MAR, the experience of infertility will still have a story, made of emotions that will need to have a place in people's lives, and this story will need to be narrated and have a space, so that it can effectively integrate into their experience.

In conclusion, support for couples is not the prerogative of this or that psychotherapeutic orientation, but it certainly must have a biopsychosocial vision that also takes into account sexuality. And it is precisely in the action of the psychosexologist that all the elements of people's lives are taken into consideration in order to build a more effective intervention.

Stefano Bernardi

Italian Center of Sexology—CIS
BolognaItalyItalian Society of Human Reproduction - SIRU
RomeItalyCIS School of Sexology
BolognaItaly

Foreword 4

The multiple facets of human infertility extend to encompass medical, social, anthropological, environmental, relational, psychological, nutritional, and technological aspects.

A dense, complex branching on which we move in the course of our profession, often following only the thickest and most robust branches, which offer us greater certainty of support.

Elena Longhi has the merit of having conceived, and subsequently realized, a book capable of providing an updated and well-organized understanding of the world of infertility, not only by gender, but also followed in the various stages of life in which such fertility can be attacked, threatened, and therefore in need of prevention as well as treatment.

The wide range of topics covered, fascinating and delicate, allows the reader to broaden his scientific horizon, contributing to form that rationality of intervention that considers the centrality of the patient as paramount, highlighting how the act of care has as its terminal the consequence that will determine on the individual or on the couple.

Furthermore, it intricately brings out the transversal concept of how in no other sector of clinical practice as in that of reproduction is the emotional, subjective and/or couple element present, and that precisely this emotional element contributes significantly to a positive result.

I am sure that this text will find significant interest and receive an excellent reception from a large number of operators active in the field of human reproduction.

Endocrinology and Andrology
CEMS (Specialist Medical Center),
Verona, Italy

Giorgio Piubello

Preface

Following volumes *Psychosexual Counseling in Andrological Surgery* and *Managing Psychosexual Consequences in Chronic Disease*, here is the completion of the trilogy with this publication on infertility from the perspective of individuals and couples, not just clinicians.

It is no coincidence that infertility has been classified as one of the most stressful situations a person can face, comparable to divorce or the death of a family member, or even to severe diseases such as neoplasms. *It is estimated that one in six couples in Western societies faces infertility in their life, and the World Health Organization has called for recognition of infertility as a global public health problem.*

In this context, the overall well-being of the couple, the success of treatment, the willingness to continue fertilization procedures, the assessment of satisfaction or dissatisfaction that people can expect due to the success or failure of treatment *are all aspects influenced by the psychological aspect of the couple.*

So Why Leave Them Alone?

<u>*And this is the premise and the ultimate goal of this discussion*</u>: Couples and single individuals are unaware of the emotional price that awaits them in any fertility therapy. The desire for a child at all costs "blinds and nullifies every other life desire," and therefore, they involuntarily exclude any preventive precaution.

Including the possibility of being accompanied by a psychosexual therapist or a specialist in human emotionality: equally complex and rich in often unexpected talents.

I like to think that these patients are unwitting therapists for a medical and psychosexual team about to ally with them.

The clinical cases, reported here in large numbers, represent only a snapshot of this varied humanity: often alone and inert in the face of not always understandable medical language, of tiring diagnostic tests, and of variables of failure or success independent of their desires.

Each of us, as a human, wants to be welcomed and listened to in our own life condition.

Also, given the fact that "we are made for some and not for all" relational, psychological, interpersonal variables often condition or favor the fertilization process.

Having a greater awareness of the value of each couple's culture can be a way to feel like "protagonists even in infertility" and not "the subordinates of clinicians."

Milan, Italy Elena Vittoria Longhi

Introduction

The term "fertility" (from the Greek "gonimótēs") appears in close connection with parent/parenthood ("goneus/gonetoitita"*), also an antonym. It describes the state of being able to have children (human beings, even animals) or provide products, seeds and fruits, but also being able to provide results such as artistic, mental, or literary works. It represents the support to creativity and productivity at a material level and also at a social, philosophical, scientific, cultural, and artistic level. Therefore, the absence of children lacks such qualities or, if present, these are imperfect, which explains why the absence of children is associated with imperfection, impotence and why it has such humiliating connotations [1].*

Infertility: The Cultural Origins

The Greek word for fatherhood ("*patrotita*") derives from the proto-Indo-European root "*ph$_2$tḗr.*" From which originates the Latin "pater." The word describes the parent, the source of origin, the one who creates, initiates, introduces, discovers, or builds and generally the one who acts in the name of God. Therefore, a father is the wise person, the leader, the inspirer, the head, and the decision-maker of the family. Also, the term stepfather ("*patrìos*") used to describe the husband of a child's mother but not the biological father of this child derives from the same root and usually takes on a negative meaning, implying the lack of wise leadership and respectful education of the child. Certainly, the absence of children from a man is not a state of honor.

In Turkish culture, there is no clear information about the use of the word "childless" ("*çocuksuz*"): perhaps in a period of unwritten oral tradition [2]. The meaning of the word child ("*çocuk*"), boy or girl in young age, means that it is in the period of development between childhood and adolescence and, metaphorically, the one who is less elderly among the elderly, a person who behaves inappropriately for the elderly, but rather a characteristic of younger people, immature and, finally, of someone who does not have sufficient experience and ability in a particular field. As seen from the definitions, the last two meanings are negative. The word child (*çocuk*) is the root of childlessness (*çocuksuzluk*) in Turkish.

In Lithuanian culture, the synonym for infertility is "*nevaisingas*," which means the one who cannot have children. This word can also mean impotence ("*impotencija*"), that is, the general incapacity and the reproductive and sexual incapacity of a man. Thus, the word parenthood ("*tėvystė*") has two meanings: being a parent and taking on the responsibilities of parents. The Lithuanian language also has separate words for fatherhood and motherhood. Fatherhood ("*tėvystė*") means being a father, the duties of the father (parents). This concept is also used when talking about a group of people who originate from a father, from a family, from a nation, etc. It could be assumed that not being a father would mean not belonging to a group or a nation. Motherhood ("*motinystė*") has three meanings. The concept describes the condition of a woman during pregnancy, childbirth, and breastfeeding; being a mother; the position of the mother, duty. Another meaning is the mother's feelings for her children and the biological relationship of the mother with her children.

In Finland, there are more meanings to define the lack of children ("*lapston*"), but there is no clear definition [3]: there are many expressions to define the "childless marriage" ("*lapseton avioliitto*") or the "couples suffering from involuntary childlessness" ("*tahattomasta lapsettomuudesta kärsivät pariskunnat*"). Also, the adjective childless ("*lappton*") refers to someone who does not have children (voluntarily or involuntarily) [4].

As noted by Heinämäki [5] in Finnish, there are two adjectives that refer to the involuntary absence of children: one that is slightly more neutral and refers to something that was not chosen or planned ("*tahaton*"), and another that refers to something that was not wanted to happen or something against one's will ("*vastentahtoinen*").

In Greece, childless women were considered sinners, bringers of bad luck, and useless (*"akliri")* (=without heirs), *"steira"* (=sterile/infertile), *"magoufa"* (=person to avoid, without family, all alone, miserable), *"marmara"* (infertile, sterile, bad), "grousuza" (bad-luck bringer), *"aneprokopi"* (=useless), *"baskani"* (=with an evil eye).

According to a study by Tarlatzis et al. [6], among infertile couples in Greece, women showed high defensive anxiety, presented psychosomatic symptoms, suffered from pre-existing guilt for abortions, and seemed to have greater difficulties in social adaptation processes. It was found that both spouses presented emotional disorders, although not severe, or had psychological problems, special needs and fears, and reported sexual dysfunctions (50% of cases) mostly associated with a certain degree of deterioration of their marriage. Finally, couples from rural areas seem to be the most burdened by traditional rules.

Infertility Yesterday and Today

Even today, infertility is perceived in a prejudiced way, so that the infertile couple are inclined to hide their problems and keep their distance from society [7]. Living without children refers to incompleteness and social exclusion [8]. Families often avoid meetings with relatives, friends, or work colleagues. But also the voluntary choice not to have children is often seen as immoral. A significant percentage of women at risk of infertility suffer from stigmatization and insults [9] and sometimes physical violence [10]. Consequently, the lack of children constitutes a gender inequality because women are perceived as selfish or judged for their inability to conceive, whereas men without children are considered interesting and are not stigmatized [11].

From these etymological premises, it is clear how much fertility professionals should understand the anguish experienced by people who turn to their practice and could be better prepared to offer them individualized support, improving relationships between doctors and patients, within the family of origin and the social network, promoting the couple's ability to live as "*unconscious therapists*" in the team of technicians.

All the more so, since although today the relationship between emotional stress and infertility has been widely accepted, this knowledge is not yet widely used in the care of the infertile couple. One of the reasons for this lies in the difficulty of attributing a clear causal relationship between infertility and emotional factors. However, the evidence of the existence of such a relationship is overwhelming. Emotional tensions can directly influence fertility by altering the hypothalamic-pituitary pathways or causing tubal spasms and indirectly contributing to vaginismus, dyspareunia, frigidity, and decreased male libido [12]. Equally important is the concept that infertility can cause emotional stress, thus starting a vicious circle. Many couples who before the development of an infertility problem (who were in a state of good emotional health) suffer from severe emotional exhaustion associating the state of infertility with an "*infertility crisis*."

This can be aggravated by infertility tests, treatments, and the therapist's instructions which invade the couple's psychosexual life. It is therefore necessary for the doctor dealing with the infertile couple to be aware:

1. *of the role of primary emotional factors in the infertility problem,*
2. *that emotional factors are created by infertility,*
3. *of the additional emotional tensions that clinical tests and treatments could add to the problem.*

Proof of this is the study by Boivin J et al. [13] which evaluated ***the impact of infertility on mental health, relationships, and daily activities for 1944 respondents***. The respondents were sterile male or female patients (n = 1037) or partners of infertile patients (n = 907; not necessarily partners of the patient sample) and were recruited at different stages of the treatment path. The most common emotions were "***sadness***" at the diagnosis of infertility and "***anxiety***" during treatment. Envy of other people who have achieved a pregnancy was often reported by women. ***More than half of the respondents (60.4%; n = 1174) perceived that the clinical path had an impact on their mental health and 44.1% (n = 857) of respondents sought mental health support.*** *A greater number of patients reported impacts on mental health (70.1%, n = 727) compared to partners (49.3%, n = 447).* Of these respondents, 55.0% (*n* = 409) strongly agreed that infertility caused emotional stress. Patients more often than partners reported a harmful impact on daily activities and "***on the balance between work and private life***." *Conversely, a disparity was found between the number of interviewees who reported mental health problems and the number of those who sought support for mental health.* This indicates the need for a multidisciplinary team to take care of the clinical, psychological, sexual, and relational aspects.

There is more. Although there is ample evidence suggesting that individual stress is continually increasing and that a high quality of the couple's relationship reduces the risk of psychological discomfort, clinicians' understanding of these factors remains limited. In the study by Yamanaka-Altenstein M et al. [14] on a sample of 116 infertile couples, *the effects of discomfort related to infertility (experienced as an individual risk factor) and the quality of the couple's relationship (experienced as a resource) were examined.*

59% of women and 23% of men reported clinical levels of psychological discomfort, 71% of women and 45% of men reported discomfort related to infertility, and 3% of participants reported a low quality of the couple's relationship.

The discomfort related to infertility predicted individual psychological discomfort, while men's discomfort related to infertility revealed psychological discomfort on the part of their partners. *Women exempt from medically assisted reproduction (MAR) treatment reported a significantly higher quality of the couple's relationship compared to women in medically assisted reproduction (MAR) treatment, and men in treatment for infertility reported significantly greater discomfort compared to non-infertile men.* The level of psychological discomfort depended on whether both or none of the partners, or only one of the partners, reported stress, anxiety and/or depression, related to infertility.

The quality of the couple's relationship was not associated with psychological discomfort, which suggests that a preliminary analysis on the couple's coping (symmetrical, conflictual, competitive, symbiotic…) could represent a useful premise for hypothesizing the reactions of each individual in situations of greater suffering.

Unfortunately, the possibility cannot be excluded of "***domestic and/or family violence on women in treatment for infertility***." The study by Çambel B et al. [15] examined the prevalence of intimate partner violence and family violence among women attending a clinic for infertility and the relationship between violence and quality of life (QoL). *The research sample consisted of 125 women who had received treatment for infertility between June and September 2019 at the Gaziantep University Hospital, Gynecology Outpatient Clinic.* The self-completed questionnaires used*:* ***Infertile Women's Exposure to Violence Determination Scale (IWEVDS), "The Fertility Quality of Life Questionnaire (FertiQoL)."***

After the diagnosis of infertility, 76.8% of women were exposed to violence. 62.5% of women stated that the perpetrator of the violence was a relative and 17.7% of them were spouses.

This once again demonstrates that infertility is a highly stressful psychological crisis for both partners, economically costly and involving complex procedures in the treatment process. Another negative effect of infertility on quality of life (QoL) is due to the resulting social pressure. These realities impact overall health levels: unhappiness, loss of expectations, and depression with low QoL. The study by Cambel B also shows a high negative correlation: ***as exposure to violence increases, the QoL of infertile women decreases, encouraging less tolerance and compliance to infertility treatment*** . It is now undeniable that infertility is a health problem with medical, psychiatric, psychological, sexual, relational, social, cultural, ethical, economic, and religious characteristics . Even if couples are not always able to evaluate all these systemic characteristics, it is the clinicians' task to organize a medical-psychosocial path, which engages the couple in every aspect of quality of life.

And what about couples waiting for infertility treatment? The study by Yamanaka-Altenstein M, et al. [16] examined 116 infertile couples. While 59% of women and 23% of men reported clinical levels of psychological distress, 71% of women and 45% of men reported distress related to infertility, and 3% of participants reported a low quality of couple relationship. Distress related to infertility predicted individual-level psychological distress ("actor effects"), while men's infertility-related distress predicted their partners' psychological distress ("partner effect"). The level of psychological distress depended on whether both, none or only one of the partners, reported distress related to infertility.

Another underestimated factor is pregnancy after infertility: Problems ended? The study by McGrath JM [17] seems to suggest the opposite. Even when infertile couples successfully give birth, they may continue to struggle with the psychological aspects of infertility and with the ongoing care of a child who may be premature, underweight at birth, or affected by another high-risk condition such as developmental or behavioral problems. Generally, positive maternal experiences progressively increase during the first year of parenthood and appear higher among ART mothers compared to mothers in the control group of various clinical studies on the subject [18]. Even compared to fathers, both the ART group and the control group showed equal attachment and care. Unpleasant birth experiences, low birth weight, and difficulty calming the baby during the first year result in high levels of parental stress in the control group, *and not among ART parents*. *Psychosexual interventions should take into account the different meanings that couples give to the history of infertility, conception, and pre- and perinatal experiences.*

What about the connection between infertility and early parent–child interactions?

A study on this by Holditch-Davis D et al. [19] examined the early parent–child interactions in infertile couples who become parents through pregnancy or adoption. Two groups of infertile couples were examined (*30 who achieved pregnancy and 21 who adopted*) and a group of 19 couples without fertility problems. The parent groups were observed interacting with their children at two moments: from 7 to 21 days after the child's birth and then a week later, in the presence of both parents. The children were aged between 9 days and 5 months. *The behaviors of the mother, father, and child were recorded every 10 s, starting when the child was picked up and ending when the child was put to sleep or an hour and a half had passed* .

No differences were found between fertile and infertile biological parents. **Adopted children** showed more alertness, less sleep, more smiles, and more observing compared to biological children. Adoptive mothers spent less time as the sole interlocutors. Adoptive parents spent more time playing with their children and held them less frequently than biological parents. ***In general, the amount of behaviors exhibited by infertile biological parents was very close to that of fertile parents.*** The differences in the behaviors of adoptive parents can be explained through the behaviors and older age of the child.

Conclusions

A diagnosis of infertility can be one of the most devastating life crises that a couple can face, leading to feelings of isolation, social stigma, and loss of control. For these reasons, psychosexual counseling is an essential component of the treatment process for both partners. In a small study [20] of 32 couples in Montreal, Quebec, couples were interviewed about their experiences with infertility and assisted reproduction technology and about their psychosocial needs during treatment. The results of this study revealed the need for patients to be informed about treatment expectations, focusing on the physical and emotional needs. Participants also emphasized the importance of having access to couple counseling and the availability of psychosexual therapists.

References

1. Gouni O, Jarašiūnaitė-Fedosejeva G, Kömürcü Akik B, Holopainen A, Calleja-Agius J (2022) Childlessness: concept analysis. Int J Environ Res Public Health 19(3):1464. https://doi.org/10.3390/ijerph19031464. PMID: 35162484; PMCID: PMC8834711
2. Yıldız N (2009) Türk destanlarında "Çocuksuzluk" ("Childlessness" in Turkish epic). Milli Folklor 21:76–88
3. Kielitoimiston Sanakirja (2020) (Dictionary of Contemporary Finnish) Helsinki: Kotimaisten Kielten Keskuksen Verkkojulkaisuja 35. Kielitoimiston Sanakirja; Helsinki, Finland. [(visited on August 18, 2021)]. URN:NBN:fi:kotus-201433
4. Childless (Senza bambini) Wikisanakirja, Free Dictionary (2021) https://fi.wiktionary.org/w/index.php?title=lapseton&oldid=4174879
5. Heinämäki E (2017) Master's thesis. University of Eastern Finland Kuopio, Finland. Omannäköiset Elämät: Lapsettomuus Keski-Ikäisten Kerrotussa

Elämänkulussa (My kind of life: the absence of children in the stories of middle-aged childless people)
6. Tarlatzis I, Tarlatzis BC, Diakogiannis I, Bontis J, Lagos S, Gavriilidou D, Mantalenakis S (1993) Psychosocial impacts of infertility on Greek couples. Hum Reprod 8:396–401. https://doi.org/10.1093/oxfordjournals.humrep.a138059
7. Drapeko N (2006) Master's thesis. Vytautas Magnus University; Kaunas, Lithuania. Nevaisingų moterų folikulinio skysčio ląstelinės sudėties ir interferono-ʏ koncentracijos tyrimas (Investigation on the cellular composition of follicular fluid and the concentration of interferon-γ in infertile women)
8. Vaitiekus E, Talačkienė D (2014) Pagalba šeimoms, negalinčioms susilaukti vaikų (Assistance to families who cannot have children). Soc Health 1:62–68
9. Papadopoulos I (2016) Endometriosis, infertility and self-stigma: results of a study on Greek and Greek-Cypriot women living in the United Kingdom. [(visited on June 2, 2021)]
10. Sabaitytė E. (2018) Master's thesis. Lithuanian University of Health Sciences; Kaunas, Lithuania:. Kūdikio susilaukti negalinčių moterų psichologinė gerovė (The psychological well-being of women suffering from infertility)
11. Šumskaitė L, Rapolienė G (2019) Motinystės diskurso paraštėse: Bevaikystė 1991–1996 m. Lietuvos moterims gonnauose žurnaluose (At the margins of the discourse on motherhood: childlessness in Lithuanian women's magazines in the period 1991–1996). Inf Sci 86:133–156. https://doi.org/10.15388/Im.2019.86.30
12. Taymor ML, Bresnick E (1979) Emotional stress and infertility. Infertility 2(1):39–47. PMID: 12339112
13. Boivin J, Vassena R, Costa M, Vegni E, Dixon M, Collura B, Markert M, Samuelsen C, Guiglotto J, Roitmann E, Domar A (2022) Tailored support may reduce mental and relational impact of infertility on infertile patients and partners. Reprod Biomed Online 44(6):1045–1054. https://doi.org/10.1016/j.rbmo.2022.01.015. Epub 2022 Feb 3. PMID: 35351377
14. Yamanaka-Altenstein M, Rauch-Anderegg V, Heinrichs N (2021) The link between infertility-related distress and psychological distress in couples awaiting fertility treatment: a dyadic approach. Hum Fertil (Camb) 25(5):924–938. https://doi.org/.1080/14647273.2021.1948112. Epub. PMID: 34232107
15. Çambel B, Akköz Çevik S (2022) Prevalence of intimate partner and family violence among women attending infertility clinic and relationship between violence and quality of life. J Obstet Gynaecol 42(6):2082–2088. https://doi.org/10.1080/01443615.2021.2024156. Epub 2022 Jan 24. PMID: 35068321
16. Yamanaka-Altenstein M, Rauch-Anderegg V, Heinrichs N (2022) The link between infertility-related distress and psychological distress in couples awaiting fertility treatment: a dyadic approach. Hum Fertil (Camb) 25(5):924–938. https://doi.org/10.1080/14647273.2021.1948112. Epub 2021 Jul 7. PMID: 34232107
17. McGrath JM, Samra HA, Zukowsky K, Baker B (2010) Parenting after infertility: issues for families and infants. MCN Am J Matern Child Nurs 35(3):156–4. https://doi.org/10.1097/NMC.0b013e3181d7657d. PMID: 20453593.

18. Repokari L, Punamäki RL, Poikkeus P, Tiitinen A, Vilska S, Unkila-Kallio L, Sinkkonen J, Almqvist F, Tulppala M (2006) Ante- and perinatal factors and child characteristics predicting parenting experience among formerly infertile couples during the child's first year: a controlled study. J Fam Psychol 20(4):670–679. https://doi.org/10.1037/0893-3200.20.4.670. PMID: 17176203
19. Holditch-Davis D, Sandelowski M, Harris BG (1998) Infertility and early parent-infant interactions. J Adv Nurs 27(5):992–1001. https://doi.org/10.1046/j.1365-2648.1998.00587.x. PMID: 9637326
20. Leggi SC, Carrier ME, Boucher ME, et al (2014) Psychosocial services for couples in infertility treatment: what couples really want. Patient Educ Acc 94(3):390–395

Elena Vittoria Longhi

Contents

Chapter 1
Identity Cards

When the body does not respond.

Infertility and sexual dysfunctions are often underestimated during a medically assisted procreation journey. However, where they exist, they can compromise not only clinical management but also the physical and psychological health of the individual and the couple. Clinicians and patients should simultaneously evaluate the couple's sexual quality, genetics, and the state of stress that the medical process entails for a prolonged time. It affects all aspects of life, questioning the couple's emotional and relational bonds. Over the years, clinical research, despite its great merits, has favored genetic techniques, risking neglecting the mental aspect of the individual and the couple.

Over the last 15 years, there has been a growing interest in the psycho-socio-relational and sexual disorders of infertile couples, which is why the European Society of Human Reproduction and Embryology (ESHRE) has decided to establish guidelines for infertility counseling. The objectives of counseling are to explore, understand, and resolve the problems arising from infertility and infertility treatment and to clarify the ways to address the problem more effectively.

The interactions between infertility and sexuality are numerous and complex. Consequently, infertility could be considered both a cause and a consequence of sexual dysfunction (SD). While organic causes of SD are not the main cause of male infertility (only 5% of causes), erectile dysfunction (ED) and ejaculation disorders are associated with increasing difficulty in conception. Moreover, SD could be secondary to the diagnosis of infertility or diagnosed during an in vitro fertilization (IVF) program.

Infertility and the issue of the global decline in male fertility is an old topic: it was first proposed in 1974 by Nelson and Bunge [1].

WHO has reaffirmed the right to physical and mental health, as coadjutants to an adequate quality of life in the individual and the couple.

E. V. Longhi, *Framing Sexual Dysfunctions and Diseases during Fertility Treatment*, https://doi.org/10.1007/978-3-031-76726-5_1

Clinical experience has shown strong stress, feelings of guilt, inadequacy, anxiety and depression, internal couple conflicts, and mechanical sexuality according to a calendar imposed by medical fertilization protocols in individuals. Aggression and resentment between spouses occur both in the case of success in fertilization practices and in the case of failure.

Men and women experience emotional fragility and often the couple cannot face the therapies, or the communication with doctors, which is often found wanting on a psychological level. We are talking about 186 million infertile individuals worldwide out of 48 million couples [1].

Most couples discover a medical cause of their infertility with great dismay, but for the remainder, unidentifiable (idiopathic) factors emerge, which are not medical clinical but psychological, couple relational.

In addition to a sperm concentration below the norm, Nelson et al. found in the study a low sperm volume and an abnormal morphology that would tend to incriminate environmental factors, genetics, lifestyles, diet, obesity, excessive use of smoking and alcohol, as well as drug use.

Women account for 40–55% of infertility cases, while men account for 20–40% [1].

In the case of women, if there has been no previous pregnancy (regardless of the outcome), it is referred to as primary infertility. On the other hand, secondary infertility is discussed thusly: infertility can be conditioned by endometriosis, reduced ovarian reserve, and polycystic ovary syndrome [2]. Conversely, male infertility mostly stems from poor sperm quality and quantity or from medical comorbidities [3] as confirmed by recent scientific literature.

This is not all.

The procedure and medical requirements condition sexual behavior and the couple's intimacy. Medical terms can be perceived as hostile and generate anxiety in infertile men, which could ultimately lead to temporary SD. Moreover, many men will consider their infertility as a loss of masculinity and virility and may suffer from low self-esteem and depression. Therefore, in infertile men, the need to identify SD and its severity is crucial before undertaking individual infertility treatment. Sexological and psychological consultations should be seriously considered during diagnostic and therapeutic stages.

We must also consider that patients are asked by clinicians to produce a sperm sample in the laboratory. Producing sperm in an in vitro fertilization clinic can be really stressful. The most common cause is anxiety and stress associated with producing a sperm sample "on demand," especially when you feel guilty and inadequate in virility. Not to mention masturbation: differently perceived depending on cultural and religious affiliation. The impact of these common cultural myths associated with autoeroticism can lead to guilt about masturbation when patients are undergoing antiretroviral therapy. As a result, an erection is not always achieved at the right time and psychogenic impotence and anejaculation are not at all rare.

The confusion between fertility, potency, and masculinity has consequences for infertile men. Generating a child is seen as a proof of masculinity and, consequently, not generating a child is experienced as a failure of virility. Therefore, it is likely that infertile men will suffer stigma with a consequent impact on potency and sexual responses.

Some men may experience impotence following the diagnosis of azoospermia: a devastating experience for a couple during infertility management. In fact, for azoospermic patients, being informed of the absence of sperm in the ejaculate has been described as "the hardest blow of their life and the worst news they had ever received." The possibility of biological paternity was perceived as non-existent and feelings of impotence and difference emerged. The advent of intracytoplasmic sperm injection (ICSI) has allowed many azoospermic men to become biological fathers using sperm obtained from testicular sperm extraction from the epididymis or testicles (TESE), leading to "a sense of repair after the previous feeling of inadequacy." But the problem arises again in the couple's intimacy: the partner often describes feelings of devaluation and inadequacy (with destructive and depressive thoughts) despite the resolving medical practice that often results in hypoactive desire or lack of attention toward the partner.

1.1 What to Do?

Men diagnosed with azoospermia can go through different stages of their life depending on the diagnosed azoospermia, which would necessitate a detailed evaluation to provide each patient with an appropriate therapeutic strategy. Indeed, sexual and psychological counseling should be offered and strongly recommended to overcome the loss of virility and masculinity that men can experience when a diagnosis of infertility or sterility is established. Especially, since his partner poorly tolerates his depression, she considers it selfish and not at all understanding of the humiliation suffered by her and by the families of origin: "Being in a relationship with an imperfect man, can other anomalies be predicted in the future? Can her life be further marked by his lack of virility?"

Intergenerational conflicts (between families of origin and the infertile couple) are not infrequent: how can it be possible to live a satisfying sexual life if the couple cannot free themselves from criticisms and judgments about his or her inadequacies? Or if parental control over medical practices becomes obsessive and invalidating?

Everything becomes more complicated if infertility is associated with debilitating chronic diseases of one of the partners.

1.2 Infertility and Chronic Diseases

Numerous studies have examined the associations between chronic diseases and a decrease in sperm parameters.

According to the WHO, the prevalence of diabetes has almost quadrupled since 2000, affecting over 400 million people worldwide [4].

Condorelli et al. [5] found that men with type 1 or type 2 diabetes mellitus had a significantly lower sperm concentration and lower progressive motility than normal. The study concluded that young patients with type 1 diabetes mellitus may have lower ejaculate volumes due to lack of epididymal contraction, while men with type 2 diabetes mellitus may show reduced sperm parameters due to inflammatory processes.

In addition to diabetes, hypertension also implies a decrease in sperm parameters.

Guo et al. [6] showed that men with hypertension had a lower sperm volume, sperm mobility, sperm count, and number of mobile sperm compared to non-hypertensive control study patients. Moreover, a recent study by Shiraishi and Matsuyama [7] evaluated a sample of over 3700 patients and found that the prevalence of comorbidities was significantly higher in infertile men compared to fertile men.

In particular, 17.8% of infertile patients were diagnosed with hypertension, while only 7.1% of fertile men shared the same diagnosis.

Furthermore, men with newly diagnosed hypertension had higher levels of total mobile sperm count after 6 months of treatment for hypertension compared to baseline and poorly treated patients. Beyond hypertension, Shiraishi and Matsuyama [7] identified hyperlipidemia, hyperuricemia, and skin diseases more common in infertile men compared to fertile men.

But there is more.

Metabolic syndrome is defined as the combination of at least three of the following factors: central obesity, hypertension, hyperglycemia, high triglycerides, and low HLD cholesterol.

Dupont et al. [8] showed that infertile men had a higher BMI (body mass index), higher fasting blood glucose levels, and lower HDL cholesterol levels compared to fertile men.

The study concluded that metabolic syndrome is a significant risk for idiopathic infertility in men.

Similarly, Chen et al. [9] highlighted that metabolic syndrome was associated with a reduced percentage of "normal" sperm morphology and reduced sperm motility.

1.3 Environmental Toxins and Lifestyle

Recent scientific literature has hypothesized that environmental toxins are one of the main factors contributing to the decline in sperm parameters: we are talking about aggressive agents such as bisphenol A (BPA), phthalates, cadmium, and triclosan.

The study by Radwan et al. [10] examined sperm samples from 315 men, concluding that exposure to BPA was associated with an increase in immature sperm, sex chromosome disomy, as well as a decrease in sperm motility.

Last but not least, the phthalates, present in consumer goods (cosmetic creams, shampoos, adhesives, paints, pesticides, various containers (including those for food and fast food), bags, cables and packaging materials), are also implicated in the decline of sperm parameters, especially in the lower progressive motility of sperm and in the fragmentation of sperm DNA.

Specifically, Barakat et al. [11] highlighted that mice exposed to phthalates before birth had smaller gonads, prostate, and seminal vesicles. In addition to this, mice exposed to phthalates in the prenatal period showed lower serum testosterone and compromised spermatogenesis. This new evidence supports the thesis that phthalates affect sperm parameters through a variety of mechanisms, conditioning the decline of sperm parameters.

Finally, triclosan (a substance with strong antibacterial properties widely used in cosmetic products, soaps, and toothpastes) is often at the base of a lower percentage of morphologically normal sperm. Not to mention cadmium, which influences the progressive motility of sperm [12].

Beyond these toxic substances, a sedentary lifestyle also has a negative effect on spermatogenesis.

A study conducted by Yuan et al. [13] found that the average sperm concentration significantly decreases over a 5-year period. The data show that the decline in sperm concentration was more evident in students compared to nonstudents. Sedentary lifestyle, stress, and lack of sleep can be possible causes of poor spermatogenic quality.

Nematollahai et al. [14] stated that mice exposed to physical exercise had a higher sperm concentration and motility compared to the control sample of sedentary mice. Finally, work stress and lack of sleep are causes of low testosterone levels and fertility [15].

Finally, the diet.

Several studies have been conducted on the excess of fatty foods and altered sperm parameters. According to the United States Department of Agriculture, the average per capita calories consumed from "added fats and oils" increased from 337 in 1970 to 562 in 2010.

The study by Crean and Senior [16] reiterated not only the negative effects of fats on sperm parameters but especially on the progressive motility, morphology, and vitality of sperm. Furthermore, a diet rich in fats was associated with smaller testicles, a lower mass of seminal vesicles, and an epididymal mass lower than body size.

But there is more.

According to WHO statistics, between 1975 and 2016 the prevalence of overweight and obesity among children and adolescents (aged between 5 and 19 years) increased from 4% to 18%.

Since then, many studies have investigated the correlation between BMI and fertility parameters. Amjad et al. [17] demonstrated that patients with high BMI showed lower levels of follicle-stimulating hormone (FSH) compared to fertile men. As for sperm quality, a correlation emerges between BMI and sperm DNA fragmentation and oxidative damage [18].

1.4 Qualitative Research Questionnaires

Clinical research has also shown that infertility is often a silent struggle that the couple experiences in total solitude. No sharing with parents, siblings, friends.

In isolation, individuals show symmetrical, critical, spiteful, depressive behaviors and often lack emotional control. The couple becomes a sounding board of resentment and love: it is not surprising that their discomfort has been compared to the mood of cancer patients at the first diagnosis [19].

In this regard, the study by Domar et al. provides an illuminating picture.

Through the administration of the Symptom Checklist 90R, the researchers recruited 149 women with infertility, 136 with chronic pain, 22 undergoing cardiac rehabilitation, 93 with cancer, 77 with hypertension, and 11 with positive status for the human immunodeficiency virus (HIV).

Infertile women showed global scores equal to patients suffering from cancer, cardiac rehabilitation, and hypertension.

Other effective questionnaires for psychological, relational, and emotional research of infertile couples can include:

1. Fertility Problem Stress (FPS-4).
2. Fertility Quality of Life [19].
3. Fertility Problem Inventory [20].
4. FPI is a self-report questionnaire that examines the impact of stress related to infertility. It provides a global score on five critical areas in infertile individuals: social concern, sexual concern, relational concern, need for parenthood, rejection of a childless lifestyle.

If we then observed the success rates of assisted reproduction technologies, we would discover that only a 25% success rate per cycle includes mothers under 35 years, after which the percentages decrease dramatically.

This means that the failure rate is about 75%, which is distressing for people who bear the heavy financial and psychological costs of these treatments [21]. Therefore, many couples do not continue the treatment when a reasonable result is not achieved.

The WHO and NICE guidelines in the United Kingdom recommend that couples be psychologically assisted in their choices and be presented with feasible goals (National Institute for Clinical Excellence (NICE), 2004).

From all the literature, it emerges that patients stop the treatment because they choose to postpone it, due to the physical and psychological burden, for relational and personal problems, for moral/ethical objections, and/or fear of negative health effects of pharmacological treatments and organizational and clinical problems. But also because they feel alone.

In clinical practice, infertile couples are often referred to the sexologist only in case of sexual dysfunctions during the treatment, poor compliance of the couple in the various processes of reproduction, or conflict with the medical team: often experienced as too scientific, poorly predisposed to understanding the sensitivity of couples.

1.5 The Most Common Sexual Dysfunctions

And what about the couple's sexuality while waiting for, during or after an assisted fertilization treatment?

It is enough to look at Table 1.1 of the American Psychiatric Association.

In a study involving 121 women diagnosed with infertility, researchers identified a prevalence of 26% of sexual dysfunctions, while in a subsequent study experts found an even higher percentage of sexual problems (61.7%) [21]. A systematic review of the literature finally concluded that women face sexual disorders more often than men when dealing with infertility [22, 23].

Most authors note that many women suffer from sexual desire disorders, arousal disorders, vaginal hydration disorders, orgasm disorders, dissatisfaction disorders, dyspareunia, and vaginismus. In men, erectile dysfunction (ED) occurs in 26 cases per 1000 men/year. The prevalence of erectile dysfunction varies from 13% to 81% in different populations. ED increases with age and shows a strong association with economic status and comorbidity conditions. It should be noted that 5% of men worldwide also suffer from orgasm disorders.

Sexual intercourse can lose spontaneity because it is solely aimed at the "procreation of a child" and is strictly limited to "fertile" days. It loses the value of play, subject to the obsession of a pregnancy [24].

And it is increasingly associated with a sense of failure, also affecting the image that the patient has of his own body and of himself.

Add to this the fact that often the medical language appears traumatizing for the couple and medical procedures can arouse a sense of anxiety and consequent temporary erectile dysfunctions, in addition to compromising male sexual identity [25].

The "timed sex" for male partners appears particularly stressful and humiliating to be degraded to the role of "sperm donors". In women, the hormonal drugs themselves and some side effects of hormonal therapy (mood swings and weight gain) can alter sexual behavior and the quality of sexuality [26].

Table 1.1 Classification of male and female sexual disorders by the American Psychiatric Association 2013

Type of disorder	Men	Women
Desire	Male hypoactive sexual desire disorder	Female sexual interest/arousal disorder
Arousal	Erectile disorder	Female sexual arousal disorder
Orgasm	Delayed ejaculation, premature ejaculation	Female orgasmic disorder, anorgasmia
Pain	Penodynia, scrotodynia	Genito-pelvic pain/penetration disorder, vaginismus

1.6 Society, Culture, Identity, and Fertility

We must also not neglect the geographical, political, religious, and cultural belonging of infertile couples.

In most non-Western countries, the lack of children is seen as a "failure," and in India, childless women are seen by society as "incomplete."

Wives usually acquire prestige in the husband's house only after achieving motherhood, otherwise they cannot boast social prestige. Lastly, motherhood is appreciated only within marriage and unmarried mothers are not accepted by Indian society.

Still in India, infertile men experience the lack of children as a defect of identity and male sexuality, especially because of the link between fertility and potency. This is associated with the fact that in some cultures, even same-sex relationships are interpreted as proof of reproductive failure [27].

The total fertility rate in India is 3.85%. In Asia the most identifiable factors influencing female infertility are hormonal or endocrine disorders, tubal abnormalities, and cervical or uterine disorders. Among males the most common cause of infertility is oligozoospermia (sperm containing too few sperm) and the inability to have an erection or intercourse with penetration.

In many cultures, however, infertility is attributed exclusively to the woman even in the presence of erectile dysfunction of the partner [27].

1.7 The Consequences of the COVID-19 Pandemic

We must not exclude the worldwide pandemic of recent years on the fertility of couples.

In fact, the COVID-19 pandemic has impacted on physical health (over 400 million people infected and about 6 million deaths worldwide in the first 2 years following the initial epidemic), mental health [28], physical exercise [25], body weight [29], academic performance [30], employment and job security [31], income and poverty [32], loneliness [33], domestic violence [34], and fertility [35], in the sense that many fertile people delayed or stopped trying to have children because of the pandemic [36].

Research has shown that lockdowns imposed constraints on people's social and intimate lives, with postponed marriages and couples who could not live together or who had no opportunity to meet and plan for the future. Probably even more important is the way couples faced and responded to the numerous stress factors associated with lockdowns and the pandemic more generally [37, 38].

Greater economic uncertainty (especially if accompanied by job loss), school closures and reduced access to childcare have all been factors that would have put families under greater pressure and could potentially have negatively influenced couple functioning [39].

1.8 Therapies for Female Infertility

Studies reveal that the incidence of sexual dysfunction is higher in infertile women compared to those with normal fertility [40].

Problems such as the negative effects of infertility treatment and pressure from family members cause stress, psychological, and physical pain [41].

The most widely accepted hypothesis in the scientific literature is that with the increase in the duration of infertility, stress increases exponentially, the sense of guilt, and the risk to one's physical and psychological health, with consequent sexual dysfunctions or abandonment of sexuality.

Few studies have explored the impact of the duration of infertility on the onset of FSD [42]. In one study, 169 infertile women were divided into three groups based on the duration of infertility: less than 2 years (Group I), 2–5 years (Group II), and 5 years and more (Group III). It was confirmed that with the prolongation of the duration of infertility, the scores of all sexual domains decreased, except for sexual satisfaction.

A larger sample is found in the study by Dong et al. [43] conducted at the Reproductive Medicine Center of Shengjing Hospital affiliated with China Medical University.

An investigation was carried out on female sexual function and on the psychological depression of patients with infertility. Seven hundred and fifteen (715) infertile patients participated in the research between September 1, 2020 and December 25, 2020.

Patients with infertility were grouped into four categories based on the duration of infertility (defined as the time elapsed from these couples' first attempt at conception to their period of infertility) [24]: ≤2 years (Group I, $n = 262$), >2 years but ≤5 years (Group II, $n = 282$), >5 years but ≤8 years (Group III, $n = 97$), and > 8 years (Group IV, $n = 74$).

The basic pathological exclusion criteria involved are as follows:

1. diabetes,
2. high blood pressure,
3. lower genital tract abnormalities,
4. genitourinary infections,
5. genital prolapse,
6. patients whose partners had severe male infertility,
7. women whose partners had been diagnosed by specialists with sexual dysfunctions,
8. presence of psychiatric conditions (which could cause sexual dysfunctions),
9. patients on therapy with drugs that affected sexual functions (e.g., selective serotonin reuptake inhibitors, as well as serotonin and norepinephrine reuptake inhibitors).

Similarly, various types of infertility were excluded, such as endometriosis [44], PCOS [45], premature ovarian failure [46], and severe male infertility [47], which would have affected sexual functions. Taking into account previous studies, women with a total FSFI score < 8 were excluded because this score implied that they did not have sufficient sexual activity [48] or had not sought intercourse.

The adopted self-administered questionnaire consisted of three parts.

The first part collected the sociodemographic characteristics of patients with infertility: age, body mass index (BMI), primary/secondary infertility, smoking status (0 = yes, 1 = no), economic level, duration of infertility, education level (0 = ≤ high school, 1 = university, 2 = university, 3 = ≥degree), alcohol consumption status (1 = usually, 2 = sometimes, 3 = rarely, 4 = never), stress in work and life (0 = very high, 1 = high, 2 = general, 3 = low, 4 = none), and frequency of physical exercise (0 = none, 1 = <1 time a week, 2 = 1 time a week, 3 = ≥2 times a week).

The second part investigated the health and sexual quality of the participants to measure the FSFI [49] and questions about the importance of sex in general, dyspareunia, possibility of orgasm in different sexual activities, and duration of intercourse and foreplay.

The third part investigated psychological depression using the Patient Health Questionnaire (PHQ-9) [50]. Each item was assigned a score on a 4-point scale from 0 to 3, with a total severity score ranging from 0 to 27. A cut-off score ≥ 10 was used to assess the presence of depression with a Cronbach's α value ranging from 0.73 to 0.95.

1. *Results*: The likelihood that patients with infertility achieved orgasm (during various sexual activities) "always or often" was found to be less than 30%, a figure much lower than that reported by patients with normal fertility [51]. This could be due to the fact that sexual intercourse is "intentionally planned" rather than instinctive and pleasurable.
2. An extremely short duration of foreplay might indicate that the partner does not experience sufficient emotional intimacy during sex, while an extremely long duration of foreplay could indicate difficulties in approach, which could affect sexual satisfaction.
3. The prolongation of infertility over time would expose patients to greater sexual dysfunctions, physically and emotionally conditioning them. Just as infertility for over 3 years significantly affects anxiety, depression, psychiatric disorders [51], eating disorders, addictions, and obsessiveness.

1.9 Conclusions

It remains to be noted that the Center for Disease Control and Prevention [52] describes infertility as the inability to conceive after adequate unprotected sexual intercourse for a year or more for women under 35 years and for 6 months or more for patients over 35 years, while men remain fertile until old age [52–55].

However, the body often follows the mind, beyond genetics. Too often, the psychologist is only consulted by an infertile couple upon their request. The psychosexual therapist appears to be a difficult figure to incorporate into the more traditionalist medical team.

"How do we screen couples? What questions can we ask couples to see if they need a sexologist? What do we need to know about their sexuality, if the couple wants a child?"

These questions respond to a rational thought that is plausible and very focused on clinical causes that do not take into account the couple's history, the sexual experience lived, the connection with the families of origin, the competition with siblings who are already parents, with facing a society that perceives the presence of a child, in a couple, as the "real family."

As if a couple does not already represent a family system in itself.

In the most experienced teams, the psychosexual therapist can identify the partners' weaknesses, hypothesize their compliance and the timing of collaboration with the medical team, prevent phases of fatigue and low investment in therapies, intuit conflicts, and family obligations of genealogical continuity. Just think about the emotional impact of a couple with a childless marriage, compared to a dyad where one of the partners was adopted or a couple with problematic sexuality. How can we not understand that their individual and shared history may give different meaning to the eventual birth of a child? And what will become of them in the event of failure?

This also falls under the responsibility of a team. And not only of the individual patients.

Treating the infertile couple with sexual dysfunction involves addressing underlying conditions such as psychogenic erectile dysfunction, low testosterone levels, Peyronie's disease in men and genito-pelvic pain/penetration disorder (GPPPD), and low sexual desire in women. Psychogenic erectile dysfunction can be successfully treated with phosphodiesterase inhibitors. A low level of testosterone is often identified in men with infertility, but testosterone therapy is contraindicated in men who are trying to conceive. Men affected by Peyronie's disease have a new therapeutic option to address penile curvature: the injection of collagenase of *Clostridium histolyticum* directly into the penile plaque. GPPPD is a broad disorder that includes vulvodynia and vaginismus and can be treated with lubricants and moisturizing creams for topical use. We must address psychosocial factors in women with low sexual desire. Flibanserin and transdermal testosterone (off-label) are new therapies for women with low sexual desire.

The impact of drugs on the couple is also a disturbing element in the relationship between the two. On the one hand, it could limit or eliminate sexual dysfunction, and on the other, it is often experienced by the couple as an additional pathological element that confirms the genetic and psychological differences of the partners.

References

1. NCDRiskFactor Collaboration (NCD-RisC) (2016) Trends in adult body-mass index in 200 countries from 1975–2014: a pooled analysis of 1698 population-based measurement studies with 19.2 million participants. Lancet 387:1377–1396
2. Penzias A, Azziz R, Bendikson K, Cedars M, Falcone T, Hansen K et al (2021) Fertility assessment of infertile women: a committee opinion. Fertil Sterile 116(5):1255–1265. https://doi.org/10.1016/j.fertnstert.2012.09.023
3. Schlegel PN, Sigman M, Collura B, De Jonge CJ, Eisenberg ML, Lamb DJ et al (2021) Diagnosis and treatment of infertility in men: AUA/ASRM guidelines part I. Fertil Steril 115(1):54–61. https://doi.org/10.1016/j.fertnstert.2020.11.015
4. World Health Organization (2016) World health organization global report on diabetes. World Health Organization, Geneva, p 88
5. Condorelli RA, La Vignera S, Mongioì LM, Alamo A, Calogero AE (2018) Diabetes mellitus and infertility: different pathophysiological effects in type 1 and type 2 on sperm function. Front Endocrinol (Lausanne) 9:268. https://doi.org/10.3389/fendo.2018.00268
6. Guo D, Li S, Behr B, Eisenberg ML (2017) Hypertension and male fertility. World J Mens Health 35(2):59–64. https://doi.org/10.5534/wjmh.2017.35.2.59
7. Shiraishi K, Matsuyama H (2018) Effects of medical comorbidity on male infertility and comorbidity treatment on spermatogenesis. Fertil Steril 110(6):1006–1011.e2. https://doi.org/10.1016/j.fertnstert.2018.07.002
8. Dupont C, Faure C, Daoud F, Gautier B, Czernichow S, Lévy R, ALIFERT collaborative group (2019) Metabolic syndrome and smoking are independent risk factors of male idiopathic infertility. Basic Clin Androl 29:9. https://doi.org/10.1186/s12610-019-0090-x
9. Chen YY, Kao TW, Peng TC, Yang HF, Wu CJ, Chen WL (2020) Metabolic syndrome and semen quality in adult population. J Diabetes 12(4):294–304. https://doi.org/10.1111/1753-0407.12995
10. Abbey A, Halman LJ, Andrews FM (1992) Psychosocial, therapeutic, and demographic predictors of stress associated with infertility. Fertil Sterile 57(1):122–128. https://doi.org/10.1016/s0015-0282(16)54787-6
11. Barakat R, Seymore T, Lin PP, Park CJ, Ko CJ (2019) Prenatal exposure to an environmentally relevant phthalate mixture disrupts testicular steroidogenesis in adult male mice. Environ Res 172:194–201. https://doi.org/10.1016/j.envres.2019.02.017
12. Nassan FL, Mínguez-Alarcón L, Williams PL, Dadd R, Petrozza JC, Ford JB, Calafat AM, Hauser R, EARTH Study Team (2019) Urinary triclosan concentrations and semen quality among men from a fertility clinic. Environ Res 177:108633. https://doi.org/10.1016/j.envres.2019.108633
13. Yuan HF, Shangguan HF, Zheng Y, Meng TQ, Xiong CL, Guan HT (2018) Decline in semen concentration of healthy Chinese adults: evidence from 9357 participants from 2010 to 2015. Asian J Androl 20(4):379–384. https://doi.org/10.4103/aja.aja_80_17
14. Nematollahai et al. (2020) Exercise in couple's infertility. Lancet. IV(67):78–80.
15. Domínguez-Salazar E, Hurtado-Alvarado G, Medina-Flores F, Dorantes J, González-Flores O, Contis-Montes de Oca A, Velázquez-Moctezuma J, Gómez-González B (2020) Chronic sleep loss disrupts blood-testis and blood-epididymis barriers, and reduces male fertility. J Sleep Res 29(3):e12907. https://doi.org/10.1111/jsr.12907
16. Crean AJ, Senior AM (2019) High-fat diets reduce male reproductive success in animal models: a systematic review and meta-analysis. Obes Rev 20:921–933
17. Amjad S, Baig M, Zahid N, Tariq S, Rehman R (2019) Association between leptin, obesity, hormonal interplay and male infertility. Andrologia 51(1):e13147. https://doi.org/10.1111/and.13147
18. Pearce KL, Hill A, Tremellen KP (2019) Obesity related metabolic endotoxemia is associated with oxidative stress and impaired sperm DNA integrity. Basic Clin Androl 29:6. https://doi.org/10.1186/s12610-019-0087-5

19. Newton CR, Sherrard W, Glavac I (1999) The fertility problem inventory: measuring perceived stress related to infertility. Fertil Sterile 72(1):54–62. https://doi.org/10.1016/S0015-0282(99)00164-8
20. Domar AD, Zuttermeister PC, Friedman R (1993) The psychological impact of infertility: a comparison with patients with other medical conditions. J Psychosom Obstet Gynaecol 14(Suppl):45–52
21. Vayena E, Rowe PJ, Griffin PD (2002) Current practices and controversies in assisted reproduction: report of a meeting on medical, ethical and social aspects of assisted reproduction, held at WHO headquarters in Geneva. World Health Organization, Geneva
22. Gameiro S, Boivin J, Peronace L, Verhaak CM (2012) Why do patients discontinue fertility treatment? A systematic review of reasons and predictors of discontinuation in fertility treatment. Hum Reprod Update 18(6):652–669. https://doi.org/10.1093/humupd/dms031. Epub 2012 Aug 6. PMID: 22869759; PMCID: PMC3461967
23. Piva I, Lo Monte G, Graziano A, Marci R (2014) A literature review on the relationship between infertility and sexual dysfunction: does fun end with baby making? Eur J Contracept Reprod Health Care 19(4):231–237. https://doi.org/10.3109/13625187.2014.919379
24. Nelson CJ, Shindel AW, Naughton CK, Ohebshalom M, Mulhall JP (2008) Prevalence and predictors of sexual problems, relationship stress, and depression in female partners of infertile couples. J Sex Med 5(8):1907–1914
25. Wischmann TH (2010) Sexual disorders in infertile couples. J Sex Med 7(5):1868–1876. https://doi.org/10.1111/j.1743-6109.2010.01717.x
26. Cousineau TM, Domar AD (2007) Psychological impact of infertility. Best Pract Res Clin Obstet Gynaecol 21:293–308. https://doi.org/10.1016/j.bpobgyn.2006.12.003
27. Ohl J, Reder F, Fernandez A, Bettahar-Lebugle K, Rongières C, Nisand I (2009) Impact of infertility and assisted reproductive techniques on sexuality. Gynecol Obstet Fertil 37:25–32. https://doi.org/10.1016/j.gyobfe.2008.08.012
28. Coëffin-Driol C, Giami A (2004) The impact of infertility and its treatments on sexual life and couple's relationship: review of the literature. Gynecol Obstet Fertil 32:624–637. https://doi.org/10.1016/j.gyobfe.2004.06.004
29. Skakkebæk A, Moore PJ, Chang S, Fedder J, Gravholt CH (2018) Quality of life in men with Klinefelter syndrome: the impact of genotype, health, socioeconomics, and sexual function. Genet Med 20(2):214–222. https://doi.org/10.1038/gim.2017.110
30. Nene UA, Coyaji K, Apte H (2005) Infertility: a label of choice in the case of sexually dysfunctional couples. Patient Educ Couns 59(3):234–238. https://doi.org/10.1016/j.pec.2005.08.005
31. Robinson E, Sutin AR, Daly M, Jones A (2022) A systematic review and meta-analysis of longitudinal cohort studies comparing mental health before and during the COVID-19 pandemic. J Affect Disorder 296:567–576
32. Stockwell S, Trott M, Tully M, Shin J, Barnett Y, Butler L, McDermott D, Schuch F, Smith L (2021) Changes in physical activity and sedentary behaviours from before to during the COVID-19 pandemic lockdown: a systematic review. BMJ Open Sport Exerc Med 7(1):e000960. https://doi.org/10.1136/bmjsem-2020-000960
33. Bakaloudi DR, Barazzoni R, Bischoff SC, Breda J, Wickramasinghe K, Chourdakis M (2022) Impact of the first COVID-19 lockdown on body weight: a combined systematic review and a meta-analysis. Clin Nutr 41(12):3046–3054. https://doi.org/10.1016/j.clnu.2021.04.015
34. König C, Frey A (2022) The impact of COVID-19-related school closures on student achievement: a meta-analysis. Educ Res Practice Issues 41(1):16–22
35. Adams-Prassl A, Boneva T, Golin M, Rauh C (2020) Inequality in the impact of the coronavirus shock: evidence from real-time surveys. J Public Econ 189:104245
36. Cantó O, Figari F, Fiorio CV, Kuypers S, Marchal S, Romaguera-de-la-Cruz M, Tasseva IV, Verbist G (2022) Welfare resilience at the onset of the COVID-19 pandemic in a selection of European countries: impact on public finance and household incomes. Rev Income Wealth 68(2):293–322

37. Bu F, Steptoe A, Fancourt D (2020) Who is lonely in isolation? Cross-cohort analysis of predictors of loneliness before and during the COVID-19 pandemic. Public Health 186:31–34
38. Piquero AR, Jennings WG, Jemison E, Kaukinen C, Knaul FM (2021) Domestic violence during the COVID-19 pandemic—evidence from a systematic review and meta-analysis. J Crim Justice 74:101806. https://doi.org/10.1016/j.jcrimjus.2021.101806
39. Aassve A, Cavalli N, Mencarini L, Plach S, Livi Bacci M (2020) The COVID-19 pandemic and human fertility. Science 369(6502):370–371
40. Emery T, Koops JC (2022) The impact of COVID-19 on fertility behaviour and intentions in a middle income country. PLoS One 17(1):e0261509. https://doi.org/10.1371/journal.pone.0261509
41. Marani M, Katul GG, Pan WK, Parolari AJ (2021) Intensity and frequency of new extreme epidemics. Proc Natl Acad Sci USA 118(35):e2105482118
42. Pietromonaco PR, Overall NC (2021) Applying relationship science to evaluate how the COVID-19 pandemic may impact couples' relationships. Am Psychol 76(3):438–450. https://doi.org/10.1037/amp0000714
43. Khademi A, Alleyassin A, Amini M, Ghaemi M (2008) Evaluation of the prevalence of sexual dysfunction in infertile couples. J Sex Med 5:1402–1410. https://doi.org/10.1111/j.1743-6109.2007.00687.x
44. Dong M, Xu X, Li Y, Wang Y, Jin Z, Tan J (2021) Impact of infertility duration on female sexual health. Reprod Biol Endocrinol 19(1):157. https://doi.org/10.1186/s12958-021-00837-7
45. Facchin F, Somigliana E, Busnelli A, Catavorello A, Barbara G, Vercellini P (2019) Infertility-related distress and female sexual function during assisted reproduction. Hum Reprod 34(6):1065–1073. https://doi.org/10.1093/humrep/dez046
46. Keskin U, Coksuer H, Gungor S, Ercan CM, Karasahin KE, Baser I (2011) Differences in the prevalence of sexual dysfunction between primary and secondary infertile women. Fertil Steril 96:1213–1217. https://doi.org/10.1016/j.fertnstert.2011.08.007
47. Hämmerli S, Kohl-Schwartz A, Imesch P, Rauchfuss M, Wölfler MM, Häberlin F, von Orelli S, Leeners B (2020) Sexual satisfaction and frequency of orgasm in women with chronic pelvic pain due to endometriosis. J Sex Med 17(12):2417–2426. https://doi.org/10.1016/j.jsxm.2020.09.001
48. Steinberg Weiss M, Roe AH, Allison KC, Dodson WC, Kris-Etherton PM, Kunselman AR, Stetter CM, Williams NI, Gnatuk CL, Estes SJ, Sarwer DB, Coutifaris C, Legro RS, Dokras A (2021) Lifestyle modifications alone or combined with hormonal contraceptives improve sexual dysfunction in women with polycystic ovary syndrome. Fertil Steril 115(2):474–482. https://doi.org/10.1016/j.fertnstert.2020.08.1396
49. Benetti-Pinto CL, Soares PM, Giraldo HP, Yela DA (2015) Role of the different sexuality domains on the sexual function of women with premature ovarian failure. J Sex Med 12(3):685–689. https://doi.org/10.1111/jsm.12743
50. Bechoua S, Hamamah S, Scalici E (2016) Male infertility: a barrier to sexuality? Andrology 4:395–403. https://doi.org/10.1111/andr.12160
51. Rosen R, Brown C, Heiman J, Leiblum S, Meston C, Shabsigh R, Ferguson D, D'Agostino R (2000) The female sexual function index (FSFI): a multidimensional self-assessment instrument for the evaluation of female sexual function. J Marital Sex Ther 26(2):191–208. https://doi.org/10.1080/009262300278597
52. Kroenke K, Spitzer RL, Williams JB (2001) The PHQ-9: validity of a measure of the severity of brief depression. J Gen Intern Med 16:606–613. https://doi.org/10.1046/j.1525-1497.2001.016009606.x
53. Petr W, Stuart B (2009) The consistency of women's couple orgasm is associated with a longer duration of penile-vaginal intercourse but not foreplay. J Sex Med 6:135–141. https://doi.org/10.1111/j.1743-6109.2008.01041.x
54. Clelia ZM, Francesca CDVM, Federica V (2018) Predictors of quality of life and psychological health in infertile couples: the moderating role of infertility duration. Qual Life Res 27:945–954. https://doi.org/10.1007/s11136-017-1781-4

55. Centers for Disease Control and Prevention. [Apr 2021]; Centers for Disease Control and Prevention (2020) 7:206–225. https://www.cdc.gov/reproductivehealth/infertility/index.htm#:%7E:text=About%206%25%20of%20married%20women,to%20term%20(impaired%20fecundity)

Chapter 2
Smoking, Alcohol, Drugs, and Male Infertility

The trend toward an increase in male reproductive disorders observed in recent years can be associated at least in part with lifestyle factors such as obesity, smoking or chewing tobacco, alcohol, and some illicit drugs such as cocaine, cannabis, and so on and exposure to extreme heat. Data on other factors such as cell phone use and stress on reproductive health require in-depth study [1].

The study by Gaur et al. [2] investigated the specific impact of alcohol and smoking on the sperm quality of male partners of couples seeking treatment for primary infertility. Sperm samples from 100 alcoholics and 100 cigarette smokers were analyzed, following WHO guidelines and compared with 100 strictly nonalcoholic and nonsmoking males for the presence of asthenozoospermia, oligozoospermia, and teratozoospermia.

Results: Only 12% of alcoholics and 6% of smokers showed normozoospermia compared to 37% of nonalcoholic and nonsmoking males. Teratozoospermia dominated in alcoholics, followed by oligozoospermia. In smokers, an overall impact of asthenozoospermia and teratozoospermia was observed, but not oligozoospermia. Light smokers predominantly showed asthenozoospermia. Chronic alcoholics and smokers showed asthenozoospermia, teratozoospermia, and oligozoospermia. This demonstrates that alcohol abuse can affect sperm morphology and production. The toxins induced by smoking mainly hinder sperm motility and seminal fluid quality. The progressive deterioration of sperm quality is linked to the increasing amount of alcohol and cigarettes consumed.

These characteristics are also found in heavy-smoking and alcohol-consuming men with idiopathic infertility. Collodel et al. [3] compared the sperm quality of two groups of men with idiopathic infertility, smokers ($n = 118$) and nonsmokers ($n = 153$). Conventional sperm analysis was performed and sperm morphology was evaluated by transmission electron microscopy (TEM). The normality values recommended by the World Health Organization guidelines were used as a control for the conventional sperm analysis and the sperm values of 25 men of proven fertility

E. V. Longhi, *Framing Sexual Dysfunctions and Diseases during Fertility Treatment*, https://doi.org/10.1007/978-3-031-76726-5_2

were used for the TEM indices. Infertile smoking and nonsmoking patients showed similar sperm parameters, although sperm motility and TEM analysis values in both groups were significantly compromised compared to controls. Smoking patients were then classified as light smokers (≥1 and ≤ 10 cigarettes/day), moderate (>10 and <20 cigarettes/day), or heavy smokers (≥20 cigarettes/day). Sperm concentration and FI were significantly ($P < 0.05$) different among the three classes of smokers considered. Comparing pairs of smoker classes, sperm concentration and FI in heavy smokers were significantly lower ($P < 0.05$) than those observed in the groups of light smokers and nonsmokers. Although the sperm quality in males with idiopathic infertility does not seem to be dramatically affected by cigarette consumption, heavy smokers show a significantly lower sperm concentration and FI [4].

Several epidemiological studies conducted on humans have reported that children born to male smokers have a higher risk of childhood tumors [5] and the existence of a significant correlation between paternal smoking and childhood cancer with emphasis on the need to focus on underlying toxicological mechanisms such as genotoxic, transcriptomic, or epigenomic effects on sperm or cord blood. Similarly, several other reports have highlighted a close connection between paternal smoking and childhood leukemia.

Congenital defects such as anorectal malformations, cardiovascular anomalies, congenital heart diseases, cleft palate, hydrocephalus, urethral stenosis, spina bifida, and reduced kidney volume have been some of the developmental anomalies observed in the offspring of paternal exposure [6].

However, the data is not very conclusive on the effects of male smoking on the outcomes of fertilization in vitro (IVF).

A comprehensive review by Mostafa [7] provided a thorough overview on cigarette smoking by men and associated anomalies in count, motility, and morphology of sperm, as well as other qualitative and quantitative measures of sperm characteristics. Male smokers present various seminal anomalies, including an increase in levels of oxidative DNA damage, breaks in the sperm DNA strand, DNA adducts, chromosomal anomalies, and decreased vitality and fertility [8].

2.1 Global Statistics [9]

Over 60% of noncommunicable diseases list smoking among the risk factors, and every year more than six million deaths result from tobacco consumption and passive smoking. Despite the growing amount of evidence supporting its deleterious effects, smoking is still a widespread phenomenon, as demonstrated by recent reports from the World Health Organization. More than a third of all adult males worldwide use tobacco [10]. Similarly, about 30% of women of reproductive age smoke cigarettes. Europe is still the leading continent in terms of tobacco consumption, while in recent years, smoking rates have gradually decreased in the United States [11].

To date, more than 4700 different chemicals have been identified in tobacco smoke, ranging from heavy metals to polycyclic aromatic hydrocarbons to mutagenic chemicals.

A significant association has been reported between the levels of lead in seminal plasma and the estimate of lifetime smoking [12]: in the same way, smoking is considered the most common source of exposure to lead and cadmium. Some metallic micronutrients involved in the pathogenesis of oxidative stress and male infertility, including arsenic and the aforementioned cadmium and lead, are commonly inhaled during the combustion of tobacco or cigarette paper [13]. These metals all have mutagenic properties and are similarly associated with an increased risk of male infertility, despite there being no significant differences in volume, concentration, and sperm motility.

But there is more.

In recent decades, alterations of sperm parameters have been observed in many studies [14]: in most of them, among smokers, alterations of morphology and a decrease in concentration, motility, and vitality have been observed. A significant decrease in sperm concentrations of current smokers compared to those who had never smoked was observed in a meta-analysis of over 2500 men from five separate studies [15]. Similarly, Kunzle et al. found a significant association between smoking and reduced sperm concentration in 2100 men presenting for a fertility evaluation [16].

The American Society of Reproductive Medicine stated in 2012 that "sperm parameters and results of sperm function tests are 22% lower in smokers compared to non-smokers" [17].

More recently, a meta-analysis study on a total of 5865 subjects concluded that moderate and heavy smokers are more likely to have a reduction in the number and motility of sperm [18].

The evidence suggests a significant role of cigarette smoking in spermatogenesis; however, the impact of smoking on male fertility still needs to be fully clarified. A preventive approach to infertility should be suggested, recommending smoking cessation and the reduction of passive smoking in both women and men.

2.2 Alcohol, Drugs, and Infertility

Clinical and experimental studies have also examined alcohol consumption as a potential risk factor for male infertility, exerting a direct effect on both testosterone metabolism and spermatogenesis.

The link between alcohol and fertility was first studied in 1985. The analysis of seminal fluid samples and hormonal evaluation of 20 men with alcohol dependence syndrome revealed a significant decrease in testosterone levels, seminal fluid volume, and sperm concentration in chronic alcoholics compared to nonalcoholic patients in the control group [19].

Subsequently, a study showed that 52.3% of heavy drinkers had partial or complete spermatogenic arrest and that the average testicular weight of heavy drinkers was significantly lower compared to that of patients in the control group [20]. Muthusami and Chinnaswamy, in 2005, found a significant increase in FSH, LH, and E2 levels in chronic alcoholics, while testosterone was significantly decreased. The volume of sperm, sperm count, motility, and the number of morphologically normal sperm were significantly decreased [21].

In 2011, a meta-analysis comprising 57 studies and 29,914 patients found a significant association between alcohol, sperm volume, sperm morphology, and sperm motility [22].

Chronic alcohol consumption seems to affect fertility more than acute alcohol consumption. Hansen et al. evaluated the association between alcohol intake in the previous 5 days, sperm quality, and reproductive hormones in a cross-sectional study conducted on 347 men [23].

Alcohol intake was associated with a deterioration of most sperm characteristics, but without a consistent dose–response pattern. There was a trend toward lower sperm characteristics with higher alcohol consumption in the previous 5 days and a hormonal shift toward a higher estradiol/testosterone ratio.

Furthermore, some authors have hypothesized that even maternal alcohol consumption during pregnancy could affect the sperm quality in male offspring. From a sample of pregnant women in a Danish study, 347 young adult sons were selected: the result? Sperm concentration decreased with increasing prenatal alcohol exposure [24].

But there is more.

The use of illicit drugs can be a significant cause of male infertility and includes the use of anabolic androgenic steroids, marijuana, opioid narcotics, cocaine, and methamphetamines. The use of these illicit drugs is common in the United States, with an annual prevalence rate for any drug consistently higher in males than in females. Anabolic androgenic steroids, marijuana, cocaine, methamphetamines, and opioids all have a negative impact on male fertility and the adverse effects on the hypothalamic–pituitary–testicular axis, sperm function, and testicular structure have been reported [25].

The study by Finelli et al. [26] highlighted that alcohol could impair male fertility by damaging the anterior pituitary gland, causing the alteration of two hormones fundamental for reproductive function, luteinizing hormone (LH) and follicle-stimulating hormone (FSH), and interfering with hormonal production in the hypothalamus.

In the testicles, alcohol could impair the function of Leydig cells, which generate the main male hormone, i.e., testosterone.

Furthermore, alcohol can induce dysfunctions of Sertoli cells, which play an essential role in the maturation of sperm.

A reduction in the volume of seminal fluid and the number of sperm in males with high alcohol consumption has been observed, as has a reduction in testosterone levels with normal values of LH, FSH, and prolactin.

Carroll et al. [27] studied the use of marijuana and its potential effects on sperm parameters in individuals undergoing treatments for infertility. Following a standard sperm evaluation conducted on 229 men, the authors concluded that the use of marijuana in high or moderate amounts had a detrimental effect on sperm morphology and motility.

The intake of cocaine during pregnancy severely affects fetal development; however, little is known about its effects on male fertility. The same applies to MDMA (Ecstasy): animal models could help understand the specific effects of both substances on male fertility. Bracken et al. [28] reported an increase in cocaine use among subjects with lower sperm count and motility; Samplaski et al. [29], more recently, suggested that higher rates of concurrent substance abuse, tobacco use, and infections among cocaine users could lead to skewed results.

Finally, Vuong et al. [30] conducted a long review of the effects of opioids on endocrine parameters and concluded that there is still not enough information on the long-term effects of opioids regarding fertility, despite solid evidence of opioid-induced hypogonadism. Recent reports suggest that both the concentration and quality of sperm can be compromised in opioid users: an increase in DNA fragmentation rates and reduced expression of catalase-like and superoxide dismutase-like activity were observed in drug-dependent men compared to healthy volunteers of the same age [31] (Fig. 2.1).

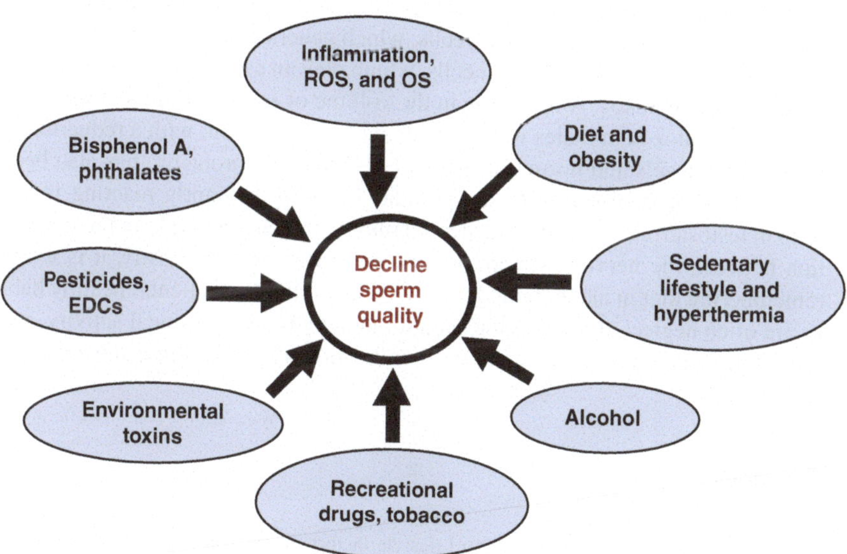

Fig. 2.1 Possible characteristics that influence sperm parameters. *IE* chemicals that alter the endocrine system, *ROS* reactive oxygen species, *OS* oxidative stress

2.3 Conclusions

Given the premises it is clear that:

1. Tobacco smoke is a mutagen of human germ cells and this could explain the potential increase in the load of genetic diseases in the offspring caused by paternal smoking, with particular attention to aneuploidy syndromes and intellectual disability, and the socioeconomic impacts of such effects. The review of the scientific literature of the last 10 years has revealed clear evidence that tobacco smoke is associated with reduced male fertility and an increase in DNA damage, aneuploidy, and sperm mutations. Studies also affirm that these effects are hereditary and have a negative impact on the offspring. A 25% increase in the frequency of sperm mutations caused by exposure to smoke inherited by the children of smokers is estimated.
2. The use of illicit drugs can be a major cause of male infertility and includes the use of anabolic androgenic steroids, marijuana, opioid narcotics, cocaine, and methamphetamines. The use of these illicit drugs is common in the United States, with an annual prevalence rate for any drug consistently higher in males than in females. Anabolic androgenic steroids, marijuana, cocaine, methamphetamines, and opioids all have a negative impact on male fertility, while adverse effects on the hypothalamus–pituitary–testicular axis on sperm function and testicular structure have been reported. The use of illicit drugs is prevalent in our society and likely has a negative impact on the fertility of men who abuse drugs.
3. Finally, the excessive and continuous use of alcohol. This substance could compromise the function of the Leydig cells, which generate testosterone. It can also induce dysfunctions of the Sertoli cells, which play an essential role in the maturation of spermatozoa. A reduction in the volume of seminal fluid and the number of spermatozoa in males with high alcohol consumption, with a reduction in testosterone levels and normal values of LH, FSH, and prolactin, has also been observed. This dysfunction of the pituitary gland in promptly reacting to the drop in testosterone suggests that alcohol plays a fundamental role in the interaction between the nervous system and the endocrine system. Lastly, it is worth remembering that in alcoholic individuals, many other fundamental healthy habits are often neglected, such as the need for healthy food or physical activity, and sometimes alcohol might be associated with smoking and/or illicit substances.

References

1. Kumar S, Kumari A, Murarka S (2009) Lifestyle factors in deteriorating male reproductive health. Indian J Exp Biol 47(8):615–624. PMID: 19775067
2. Gaur DS, Talekar MS, Pathak VP (2010) Alcohol intake and cigarette smoking: impact of two major lifestyle factors on male fertility. Indian J Pathol Microbiol 53(1):35–40. https://doi.org/10.4103/0377-4929.59180. PMID: 20090219

3. Collodel G, Capitani S, Pammolli A, Giannerini V, Geminiani M, Moretti E (2010) Semen quality of male idiopathic infertile smokers and nonsmokers: an ultrastructural study. J Androl 31(2):108–113. https://doi.org/10.2164/jandrol.109.007773. Epub 2009 Sep 10. PMID: 19745220
4. Esakky P, Moley KH (2016) Paternal smoking and germ cell death: a mechanistic link to the effects of cigarette smoke on spermatogenesis and possible long-term sequelae in offspring. Mol Cell Endocrinol 435:85–93. https://doi.org/10.1016/j.mce.2016.07.015
5. Lee KM, Ward MH, Han S (2009) Paternal smoking, genetic polymorphisms in CYP1A1 and risk of childhood leukemia. Leuk Res 33:250–258
6. Axelsson J, Rylander L, Rignell-Hydbom A, Silfver KA, Stenqvist A, Giwercmanet A (2013) The impact of paternal and maternal smoking on the quality of sperm in adolescent men. PLoS One 8(6):e66766
7. Mostafa M (2010) Cigarette smoke and male infertility. J Adv Res 1:179–186
8. Godschalk RWL, Verhofstad N, Verheijea M, Yauk CL, Linschooten JO, van Steeg H, van Oostrom CT, van Benthem J, van Schooten FJ (2015) Effects of benzo[a]pyrene on mouse germ cells: inherited DNA mutation, hypomethylation of testicular cells and their interaction with nucleotide excision repair. Toxicol Res 4:718–724
9. Sansone A, Di Dato C, de Angelis C, Menafra D, Pozza C, Pivonello R, Isidori A, Gianfrilli D (2018) Smoke, alcohol and drug addiction and male fertility. Reprod Biol Endocrinol 16(1):3. https://doi.org/10.1186/s12958-018-0320-7
10. Prevalence of tobacco consumption. http://www.who.int/topics/tobacco/en/
11. Sharma R, Harlev A, Agarwal A, Esteves SC (2016) Cigarette smoke and sperm quality: a new meta-analysis examining the effect of the 2010 World Health Organization Laboratory methods for the examination of human sperm. Eur Urol 70(4):635–645. https://doi.org/10.1016/j.eururo.2016.04.010
12. Benoff S, Centola GM, Millan C, Napolitano B, Marmar JL, Hurley IR (2003) Increased levels of lead in seminal plasma affect negatively on the fertility potential of spermatozoa in in vitro fertilization. Hum Reprod 18(2):374–383. https://doi.org/10.1093/humrep/deg020
13. Jurasovic J, Cvitkovic P, Pizent A, Colak B, Telisman S (2004) Sperm quality and reproductive endocrine function with regard to blood cadmium in Croatian male subjects. Biometals 17(6):735–743. https://doi.org/10.1007/s10534-004-1689-7
14. Asare-Anane H, Bannison SB, Ofori EK, Ateko RO, Bawah AT, Amanquah SD, Oppong SY, Gandau BB, Ziem JB (2016) Tobacco smoking is associated with a decrease in sperm quality. Reprod Health 13(1):90. https://doi.org/10.1186/s12978-016-0207-z
15. Ramlau-Hansen CH, Thulstrup AM, Aggerholm AS, Jensen MS, Toft G, Bonde JP (2007) Is smoking a risk factor for decreased sperm quality? A cross-sectional analysis. Hum Reprod 22(1):188–196. https://doi.org/10.1093/humrep/del364
16. Kunzle R, Mueller MD, Hanggi W, Birkhauser MH, Drescher H, Bersinger NA (2003) Sperm quality of smokers and non-smokers in infertile couples. Fertil Steril 79(2):287–291. https://doi.org/10.1016/S0015-0282(02)04664-2
17. Practice Committee of the American Society for Reproductive M (2012) Smoking and infertility: a committee opinion. Fertil Steril 98(6):1400–1406. https://doi.org/10.1016/j.fertnstert.2012.07.1146
18. Sharma R, Harlev A, Agarwal A, Esteves SC (2016) Cigarette smoking and sperm quality: a new meta-analysis examining the effect of the 2010 World Health Organization Laboratory methods for the examination of human semen. Eur Urol 70(4):635–645. https://doi.org/10.1016/j.eururo.2016.04.010
19. Kucheria K, Saxena R, Mohan D (1985) Sperm analysis in alcohol dependence syndrome. Andrologia 17(6):558–563. https://doi.org/10.1111/j.1439-0272.1985.tb01714.x
20. Pajarinen JT, Karhunen PJ (1994) Spermatogenic arrest and Sertoli cell-only syndrome: common human testicular disorders induced by alcohol. Int J Androl 17(6):292–299. https://doi.org/10.1111/j.1365-2605.1994.tb01259.x

21. Muthusami KR, Chinnaswamy P (2005) Effect of chronic alcoholism on male fertility hormones and semen quality. Fertil Sterile 84(4):919–924. https://doi.org/10.1016/j.fertnstert.2005.04.025
22. Li Y, Lin H, Li Y, Cao J (2011) Association between socio-psycho-behavioral factors and male semen quality: systematic review and meta-analysis. Fertil Sterile 95(1):116–123. https://doi.org/10.1016/j.fertnstert.2010.06.031
23. Hansen ML, Thulstrup AM, Bonde JP, Olsen J, Hakonsen LB, Ramlau-Hansen CH (2012) Does last week's alcohol intake affect semen quality or reproductive hormones? A cross-sectional study among healthy young Danish men. Reprod Toxicol 34(3):457–462. https://doi.org/10.1016/j.reprotox.2012.06.004
24. Ramlau-Hansen CH, Toft G, Jensen MS, Strandberg-Larsen K, Hansen ML, Olsen J (2010) Maternal alcohol consumption during pregnancy and semen quality in the male offspring: two decades of follow-up. Hum Reprod 25(9):2340–2345. https://doi.org/10.1093/humrep/deq140
25. Fronczak CM, Kim ED, Barqawi AB (2012) The insults of illicit drug use on male fertility. J Androl 33(4):515–528. https://doi.org/10.2164/jandrol.110.011874. PMID: 21799144
26. Finelli R, Mottola F, Agarwal A (2021) Impact of alcohol consumption on male fertility potential: a narrative review. Int J Environ Res Public Health 19:328. https://doi.org/10.3390/ijerph19010328
27. Payne KS, Mazur DJ, Hotaling JM, Pastuszak AW (2019) Cannabis and male fertility: a systematic review. J Urol 202:674–681. https://doi.org/10.1097/JU.0000000000000248
28. Bracken MB, Eskenazi B, Sachse K, McSharry JE, Hellenbrand K, Leo-Summers L (1990) Association of cocaine use with concentration, motility and morphology of sperm. Fertil Sterile 53(2):315–322. https://doi.org/10.1016/S0015-0282(16)53288-9
29. Samplaski MK, Bachir BG, Lo KC, Grober ED, Lau S, Jarvi KA (2015) Cocaine use in the male infertility population: an indicator of conditions leading to subfertility. Curr Urol 8(1):38–42. https://doi.org/10.1159/000365687
30. Vuong C, Van Uum SH, O'Dell LE, Lutfy K, Friedman TC (2010) The effects of opioids and opioid analogs on animal and human endocrine systems. Endocr Rev 31(1):98–132. https://doi.org/10.1210/er.2009-0009
31. Safarinejad MR, Asgari SA, Farshi A, Ghaedi G, Kolahi AA, Iravani S, Khoshdel AR (2013) The effects of opiate consumption on serum levels of reproductive hormones, on sperm parameters, on the antioxidant capacity of seminal plasma, and on sperm DNA integrity. Reprod Toxicol 36:18–23. https://doi.org/10.1016/j.reprotox.2012.11.010

Chapter 3
Infertility and Cancer

The consequences of treatments in children, adolescents, adults: What sexuality?

Most of the literature regarding adolescent reproductive health has focused on the prevention of sexually transmitted infections and unwanted pregnancies.

A topic rarely considered in the care of children and adolescents is *fertility*.

Adolescents and young adults (AYA) diagnosed with cancer and undergoing treatment are at risk of having harmful effects on their psychosocial maturation, sexual behavior, identity development, and intimate relationships. Cancer-related sexual dysfunction is caused by a combination of physiological changes induced by cancer and its treatment (surgery, radiotherapy, and chemotherapy). Surgery, depending on the amount of tissue or organ removed, and radiation can cause changes to nerves and blood vessels in the genital area. Such changes can cause erectile dysfunction and ejaculation problems in men and affect sexual sensitivity (both desire and orgasm) in women and men. Chemotherapy can affect the hormones that control normal sexual function.

Changes in hormone levels can cause symptoms of early menopause in women, including vaginal dryness, narrowing, and loss of elasticity. The extent of these problems and the resulting psychosocial challenges that accompany sexual problems are not well understood for this age group. Early complications of treatment such as fatigue and nausea can hinder intimacy and interest in sexual activity.

Late effects can include unfavorable changes in self-esteem and body image, as well as physical complications and symptoms that can have lasting effects on sexual performance.

Oncological therapy (including chemotherapy and radiotherapy), bone marrow transplantation for malignant and nonmalignant conditions, and alkylating agents used for treatments are causes of infertility and presuppose a separate project.

In addition, rheumatic and renal conditions, hormonal therapy used among young transgender people, sexual development disorders, and other genetic syndromes such as cystic fibrosis and galactosemia have an impact on fertility.

E. V. Longhi, *Framing Sexual Dysfunctions and Diseases during Fertility Treatment*, https://doi.org/10.1007/978-3-031-76726-5_3

It is estimated that about 6.7 million women and 3.3–4.7 million men in the United States have fertility problems.

Likewise, almost 15% of the male population in the United States is affected by some form of infertility, with rates reaching 35–55% among male survivors of childhood cancer.

Adolescents and young adults (AYA) faced with potential infertility following gonadotoxic treatments have reported discomfort and impairment of quality of life, both at the time of diagnosis and following therapeutic treatments.

In fact, infertility has been identified as one of the major factors contributing to marital disagreements and is one of the main causes of depression in adults.

Meanwhile, assisted reproduction technologies have been developed to preserve gametes for future use, including the cryopreservation of sperm for pubertal males and the cryopreservation of oocytes for postmenarcheal females. Experimental research has also examined the preservation of testicular and ovarian tissue for prepubertal males and premenarchal females.

The American Academy of Pediatrics, the American Society of Clinical Oncology, and the American Society for Reproductive Medicine have urged clinicians to discuss potential infertility with at-risk patients before starting treatment and to offer them timely methods for preserving fertility.

Among the fertility preservation methods available to pediatric patients, sperm banking is the least invasive (with samples usually collected through masturbation); however, *financial constraints and the ethical, social, and religious concerns of clinicians and families prevent widespread use of this technology.*

It should be noted that numerous studies have shown the following:

- many groups of pediatric practitioners feel inadequately trained in this area;
- sperm banking counseling practices vary depending on the Reference Clinical Centers;
- the AYA bank has a minimum amount of sperm.

Many AYA males (who have not preserved sperm) later report having received insufficient information about sperm banking and therefore express regret for this missed opportunity.

A study completed by Cherven et al. [1] in eight different pediatric oncology centers shows that male adolescents who have just been diagnosed with cancer were more likely to consider sperm banking provided that the reference clinicians (mostly pediatric oncologists) were comfortable discussing the topic with them.

Clinical experience shows that even teenagers perceive clinicians' discomfort in discussing the risk of infertility and the process of sperm preservation. In this sense, there is still much to do in deepening the communicative style and the positive connotation in the doctor–patient–family relationship.

But there is more.

3.1 Oncofertility

Clinical research [2] has shown that 1 in 29 men under the age of 50 developed invasive cancer between 2009 and 2011.

Meanwhile, 5-year survival rates for most cancers have significantly improved and consequently, there has been an increased demand for parenthood from male cancer survivors of reproductive age.

It is well known that chemotherapy, conditioning regimens for bone marrow transplantation, or alkylating agents, can compromise fertility [3]. In Western countries, there is a trend to delay childbirth [4], with male partners seeking fatherhood at an older age. It is therefore desirable that the needs for fertility preservation in young male cancer patients will be met over time [5].

The American Society of Clinical Oncology (ASCO) updated its guidelines in 2013 (initially drafted in 2006), recommending that practitioners discuss fertility preservation with all patients of reproductive age who will receive treatment carrying a possible risk of iatrogenic infertility. It is recommended that sperm be obtained before the start of gonadotoxic treatment [6].

Schover et al. [7] conducted a study on men aged between 14 and 40 years, demonstrating that about half of the men with cancer were interested in having children in the future, including 77% of men who did not yet have children at the time of diagnosis.

Among the men interviewed in this retrospective study, only 51% remembered being offered sperm preservation and 24% reported having preserved their sperm.

The most common reason given by patients who did not preserve their sperm in a bank was insufficient information (no counseling or the occurrence of unanswered questions) received.

Other studies on the subject are as follows:

Chong et al. [8] conducted two studies on pediatric patients and showed a sperm bank incidence of less than 30% [9].

Although numerous reports have been published on fertility counseling rates and sperm banks, most studies include a single type of cancer, mainly focus on pediatric patients or incorporate data from surveys [10].

Grover et al. [11] used the UNC (University of North Carolina) tumor registry to identify all men aged between 13 and 50 years who were diagnosed with cancer between January 1, 2013 and May 1, 2015.

742 male patients aged between 13 and 50 years with a new cancer diagnosis between January 1, 2013 and May 1, 2015 were recruited.

Of these, 541 patients were excluded because they were exempt from chemotherapy treatment, leaving 201 patients for the study.

Other reasons for exclusion included receiving chemotherapy outside of UNC (60 patients), receiving palliative chemotherapy (51 patients), history of previous cancer or chemotherapy outside of the time frame (nine patients), history of vasectomy (seven patients), and mental retardation/developmental delay (two patients).

Most of the participated patients were white, over 30 years old, unmarried, and had no children.

Of the 201 men included in the study, only 29% (59 patients) were informed about fertility-related risks.

Of the 59 patients who requested counseling, 39% (23 patients) attempted to preserve their sperm (11% of the entire cohort) and of these patients, 87% (20/23 patients) successfully preserved it. Overall, only 10% successfully collected sperm before the start of chemotherapy.

Interest in sperm preservation seems to be very high at all ages, as shown by:

1. a 15-year retrospective study [12] on cancer patients referred to the sperm bank at a French center, in which the average age of the sperm bank donor was 29.3 years, with an age range from 12.7 to 64.8 years.
2. a retrospective study [13] on patients suffering from cancer who preserved their sperm in a Brazilian center, the average age was 33 years, with an age range between 16 and 69 years.

On the other hand [10], in a recently published study involving a questionnaire administered to 200 men with testicular cancer, 70% of patients reported having decided not to preserve their sperm, due to lack of interest (51%) and time constraints (18%). Seventeen percent of patients in the study did not deposit their sperm because this option was not offered to them, and another 9% did not perform the collection due to costs.

3.2 Young Adults and Infertility

Statistical studies [14] indicate that there are about 500,000 childhood cancer survivors living in the United States, many of whom may be at risk of infertility related to cancer treatment [15].

As part of cancer treatment, children and adolescents are often exposed to gonadotoxic therapies (e.g., heavy metal chemotherapy or alkylating, radiation and/or surgical interventions on the gonads, hematopoietic stem cell transplant), which are associated with premature or primary ovarian failure [16], failure in females, and oligospermia or azoospermia in males.

Compared to their siblings, cancer survivors, both male and female, run a higher risk of infertility.

We must not forget that fertility-related concerns are associated with psychological distress, depression, and anxiety, particularly for younger survivors and those without children.

As a matter of fact, the study by Armuand et al. [17] identified 810 cancer survivors between 2003 and 2007 aged between 18 and 45 years (taken from national registries). A postal questionnaire was sent including specific questions for the study, Short-Form 36 Health Survey and the Fertility Problem Inventory, the response was 60% with 484 questionnaires completed and returned.

Results: Patients who wanted to have children at the time of cancer treatment were more likely to receive fertility-related information and to be referred to a fertility clinic for FP [18].

However, since qualitative studies conducted on young adult cancer survivors indicate that patients may change their minds about future children [19], there is a risk that some patients, who refuse FP because they do not want children at the time of treatment, may reconsider the decision later [20].

In any event, there is no doubt that fertility-related concerns can have a negative impact on self-confidence and body image [21]. Survivors may fear that infertility could have a negative impact on their desirability as a partner and on future romantic relationships, perceiving imminent criticism from parents and in-laws if they did not pursue biological parenthood.

Women cancer survivors who were diagnosed in adolescence report greater fertility-related distress than male survivors: they report feeling upset, nervous, overwhelmed, and restless (especially in the context of uncertain fertility), they express greater concerns about their partner's reactions, and they experience obsessive thoughts about possible or unlikely fertility [22].

Survivors also claim to have received little information after treatment about their fertility potential and treatment options. Moreover, most childless cancer survivors desire [22] biological parenthood. When this is not possible, some survivors [23] experience even greater discomfort due to perceived health-related discrimination and/or the high financial costs associated with the adoption or surrogacy process.

Not to mention that among the concerns of these patients of both genders are: the heredity of the cancer pathology and the fear of recurrence.

In women, there is also the concern of carrying a pregnancy to term and being the cause of cardiac, respiratory, weight-related complications for the fetus during pregnancy. On the other hand, a decrease in fertility-related problems has been reported in those who have undergone fertility preservation.

Unfortunately, there are significant obstacles to fertility preservation for children and adolescents undergoing cancer treatment, and uptake remains limited [24].

3.3 What about the Sexuality of the Couple?

Examining sexual functioning and sexual satisfaction as additional aspects of sexuality, some studies have described a greater sexual dysfunction and less sexual satisfaction [25, 26] in CCS compared to references. Greater problems with sexual functioning have been reported by female CCS [27]. Moreover, previous studies have reported that worse sexual functioning is associated with survivors' level of discomfort, a lower quality of life (QoL) related to health, health problems, fatigue, infertility, negative perception of one's body and scars [28]. It has been shown that similar factors are associated with a decrease in sexual satisfaction, namely the absence of a partner, survival from central nervous system cancer, as well as the experience of fertility problems and body dissatisfaction. The study by Wettergren [26] examined the impact of cancer on sexual function and intimate relationships in adolescents and young adults (AYA).

The participants (*n* = 465, ages 15–39) in the study Adolescent and Young Adult Health Outcomes and Patient Experience (AYA HOPE) completed two surveys about 1 and 2 years after the cancer diagnosis. Forty-nine percent of AYAs reported negative effects on sexual function 1 year after the cancer diagnosis and 70% of these persisted in their negative perceptions 2 years after the diagnosis. Those who reported a negative impact at 2 years were more likely to be 25 years or older (OR, 2.53; 95% CI, 1.44–4.42), not have children (OR, 1.81; 95% CI, 1.06–3.08), and reported that their diagnosis had a negative effect on physical appearance (OR, 3.08; 95% CI, 1.97–4.81).

The most common problems reported include pain, lack of desire, lack of orgasm, and arousal difficulties [29]. Furthermore, women may be troubled by vaginal dryness and men may suffer from erectile and ejaculatory dysfunction. It is difficult to determine the prevalence of sexual dysfunction among those diagnosed with AYA (ages 15–39 years) because the available data combine the results with younger populations.

The sexual health conditions that affect young women during or after cancer treatment can be considered according to the same categories of female sexual dysfunctions in the general population. The American Psychiatric Association defines the following female sexual disorders: sexual interest/arousal, orgasm, and genito-pelvic pain/penetration [30].

Once active cancer treatment is completed, young patients should be screened for sexual health problems. Dysfunctions in this area are common among those who complete treatment and, although most disorders can be treated, opportunities to address them are often missed. In a follow-up study of patients after pelvic radiotherapy, sexual problems were addressed in only 25% of visits [31].

When addressing sexual function, it is essential not to make assumptions about sexual orientation or sexual practices.

The young patient should be asked open-ended questions that allow them to feel comfortable sharing information relevant to their evaluation and management. Many young people, men and women, who have already had relationships with same-sex peers, often feel excluded from clinical interest or excluded from a sexual anamnesis intended exclusively for heterosexuals. Young couples also often feel accompanied in the oncological journey but not with regard to their quality of life: including sexuality and especially in individual and/or couple experiences.

Certainly, there are obstacles in addressing sexual health problems, including time constraints or a reluctance by doctors to even raise sexual health issues, and the feeling that many women may feel embarrassed to ask for information about these problems or may not be aware of the availability of treatment. Young male patients are not accustomed to talking about their sexuality: especially with male doctors because the competition between the "healthy" clinician and the young man with probable sexual dysfunctions, in the here-and-now and in the future, becomes unmanageable.

Furthermore, some patients may fear that their oncologist perceives these problems as trivial or that the patient is ungrateful for their care. However, questions about sexual health can be formulated in a neutral way and incorporated into a further routine review posttreatment. In addition to asking these questions, it is important to ensure that resources are available locally for patients who wish to continue treatment [32].

Sexuality is an important aspect of life and is often affected in patients diagnosed with cancer. For women, estimates of sexual dysfunction range from 40% to 100%. The New England Association of Gynecologic Oncologists (NEAGO) conducted a survey among gynecologic oncologists about any reservations in conducting a sexual anamnesis on cancer patients [33]. Although almost all respondents claimed to be comfortable addressing the sexual problems of their patients, less than half collected a sexual anamnesis in new patients and 80% did not believe there was enough time to devote to exploring sexual issues. The further results of this survey suggest that aspects of sexual dysfunction in women with gynecological cancer may be overlooked by gynecological oncology practitioners. This prompts cancer programs to develop formal resources for women with questions about sexuality following a cancer diagnosis.

Young male patients are often assisted by family members who consider an investigation into sexual development and practice unnecessary, often denying the problem. This will lead to the young adult experiencing certain sexual dissatisfaction, leading, in the most evident cases, to avoiding encounters with partners or to isolating themselves in a disappointing autoerotic practice, not without feelings of guilt.

3.4 Conclusions

Fertility preservation may not be feasible also due to fears related to the invasiveness of procedures, high costs, timing, and delays in starting treatment. To family beliefs, to the culture of origin, to the religion to which they belong. However, clinicians have a role as facilitators of medical and relational processes: educating young patients and their families represents an investment in future life projects and a conservative methodology. It is certain that in addition to the clinical field, sexual education should open paths of reflection not only on male and female sexual response and sexually transmitted diseases but also on the preservation and quality of male and female fertility.

We must consider that among the methods of fertility preservation available to pediatric patients, the sperm bank is the least invasive (with samples usually collected through masturbation) and has been used effectively for decades; however, barriers such as financial constraints and ethical, social, and religious concerns of providers and families prevent widespread use of this technology.

Note that numerous studies have shown that:

1. many groups of pediatric providers feel inadequately trained in this area;
2. sperm banking counseling practices are variable among providers and centers, and a minority of AYA bank sperm;
3. many AYA males who did not bank sperm later report having received insufficient information about the bank and therefore express regret for this missed opportunity.

A study completed by Klosky et al. [25] at eight different pediatric oncology centers shows that male adolescents who have just been diagnosed with cancer were more likely to use the sperm bank if pediatric oncologists were complicit and reassuring about the conservative practice. Furthermore, patients who turned to fertility specialists were five times more likely to preserve their semen. This is because they are more prepared for sexual dysfunctions to which they would be more exposed in the present and in adulthood. Being men often becomes a denied possibility for these boys, an insurmountable difference, a conditioning in planning a future for two. These results are consistent with previous literature, showing the positive impact of standardizing counseling practices on semen bank rates. In particular, Klosky et al. wish to show that teenagers are dependent on and conditioned by the personal attitude of pediatric oncologists depending on whether they appear hesitant, morally uncertain, or affable and reassuring. Given that this discomfort is associated with lower rates in semen banks, these data strongly suggest that providers involved in the care of patients at risk of infertility should receive training in this area and/or should direct specialists who feel comfortable guiding a patient and a family through the semen banking process. In addition to accompanying them on an educational journey to sexuality even following a disabling disease.

References

1. Cherven B, Kelling E, Lewis RW, Pruett M, Meacham L, Klosky JL (2022) Fertility-related worry among emerging adult cancer survivors. J Assist Reprod Genet 39(12):2857–2864. https://doi.org/10.1007/s10815-022-02663-1
2. Siegel RL, Miller KD, Jemal A (2015) Cancer statistics. CA Cancer J Clin 65:5–29
3. Ethics Committee of the American Society for Reproductive Medicine (2013) Fertility preservation and reproduction in patients undergoing gonadotoxic therapies: committee opinion. Fertil Steril 100:1224–1231
4. Wallace WH, Anderson RA, Irvine DS (2005) Fertility preservation for young patients with cancer: who is at risk and what can be offered? Lancet Oncol 6:209–218
5. Salonia A, Matloob R, Saccà A et al (2012) Are Caucasian-European men delaying fatherhood? Results of a 7-year observational study on infertile couples with male factor infertility. Int J Androl 35:125–132
6. Lee SJ, Schover LR, Partridge AH, Patrizio P, Wallace WH, Hagerty K, Beck LN, Brennan LV, Oktay K, American Society of Clinical Oncology (2006) American Society of Clinical Oncology recommendations on fertility preservation in cancer patients. J Clin Oncol 24(18):2917–2931. https://doi.org/10.1200/JCO.2006.06.5888. Epub 2006 May 1. Erratum in: J Clin Oncol. 2006; 24(36):5790

7. Schover LR, Brey K, Lichtin A, Lipshultz LI, Jeha S (2002) Knowledge and experience regarding cancer, infertility, and sperm banking in younger male survivors. J Clin Oncol 20(7):1880–1889. https://doi.org/10.1200/JCO.2002.07.175
8. Chong AL, Gupta A, Punnett A, Nathan PC (2010) A cross Canada survey of sperm banking practices in pediatric oncology centers. Pediatr Blood Cancer 55(7):1356–1361. https://doi.org/10.1002/pbc.22705
9. Klosky JL, Randolph ME, Navid F, Gamble HL, Spunt SL, Metzger ML, Daw N, Morris EB, Hudson MM (2009) Sperm cryopreservation practices among adolescent cancer patients at risk for infertility. Pediatr Hematol Oncol 26(4):252–260. https://doi.org/10.1080/08880010902901294
10. Sonnenburg DW, Brames MJ, Case-Eads S, Einhorn LH (2015) Utilization of sperm banking and barriers to its use in testicular cancer patients. Support Care Cancer 23(9):2763–2768. https://doi.org/10.1007/s00520-015-2641-9
11. Grover NS, Deal AM, Wood WA, Mersereau JE (2016) Young cancer patients experience low referral rates for fertility counseling and sperm banking. J Oncol Pract 12(5):465–471
12. Bizet P, Saias-Magnan J, Jouve E et al (2012) Sperm cryopreservation before cancer treatment: a 15-year single-center experience. Reprod Biomed Online 24:321–330
13. Bonetti TC, Pasqualotto FF, Queiroz P, Iaconelli A Jr, Borges E Jr (2009) Sperm banking for male cancer patients: social and semen profiles. Int Braz J Urol 35(2):190–197; discussion 197–198. https://doi.org/10.1590/s1677-55382009000200009
14. Howlader N, Noone AM, Krapcho M, Miller D, Brest A, Yu M, Ruhl J, Tatalovich Z, Mariotto A, Lewis DR, Chen HS, Feuer EJ, Cronin KA (eds) (2021) SEER cancer statistics review, 1975–2018. National Cancer Institute, Bethesda
15. Hudson MM, Ness KK, Gurney JG, Mulrooney DA, Chemaitilly W, Krull KR, Green DM, Armstrong GT, Nottage KA, Jones KE, Sklar CA, Srivastava DK, Robison LL (2013) Clinical ascertainment of health outcomes among adults treated for childhood cancer. JAMA 309(22):2371–2381. https://doi.org/10.1001/jama.2013.6296. Erratum in: JAMA 2013; 310(1):99
16. Green DM, Kawashima T, Stovall M, Leisenring W, Sklar CA, Mertens AC, Donaldson SS, Byrne J, Robison LL (2010) Fertility of male survivors of childhood cancer: a report from the childhood cancer survivor study. J Clin Oncol 28(2):332–339. https://doi.org/10.1200/JCO.2009.24.9037
17. Armuand GM, Wettergren L, Rodriguez-Wallberg KA, Lampic C (2014) Desire for children, difficulties achieving a pregnancy, and infertility distress 3 to 7 years after cancer diagnosis. Support Care Cancer 22(10):2805–2812. https://doi.org/10.1007/s00520-014-2279-z
18. Adams E, Hill E, Watson E (2013) Fertility preservation in cancer survivors: a national survey of oncologists' current knowledge, practice and attitudes. Br J Cancer 108(8):1602–1615. https://doi.org/10.1038/bjc.2013.139
19. Carter J, Lewin S, Abu-Rustum N, Sonoda Y (2007) Reproductive issues in the gynecologic cancer patient. Oncology (Williston Park) 21(5):598–606
20. Connell S, Patterson C, Newman B (2006) A qualitative analysis of the reproductive issues raised by young Australian women with breast cancer. Int Women's Health 94(1):94–110. https://doi.org/10.1080/07399330500377580
21. Benedetto C, Shuk E, Ford JS (2016) Fertility issues in adolescents and young adults who survived cancer. J Adolesc Young Adult Oncol 5(1):48–57. https://doi.org/10.1089/jayao.2015.0024
22. Schover LR (2005) Motivation for parenthood after cancer: a review. J Natl Cancer Inst Monogr 34:2–5. https://doi.org/10.1093/jncimonographs/lgi010
23. Gorman JR, Whitcomb BW, Standridge D, Malcarne VL, Romero SA, Roberts SA, Su HI (2017) Adoption consideration and concerns among young adult female cancer survivors. J Cancer Surviv 11(1):149–157. https://doi.org/10.1007/s11764-016-0572-1

24. Bartolo A, Santos IM, Monteiro S (2021) Towards an understanding of the factors associated with reproductive concerns in younger women cancer patients: evidence from the literature. Oncol Nurses 44(5):398–410
25. Klosky JL, Anderson LE, Russell KM, Huang L, Zhang H, Schover LR, Simmons JL, Kutteh WH (2017) Provider influences on sperm banking outcomes among adolescent males newly diagnosed with cancer. J Adolesc Health 60(3):277–283. https://doi.org/10.1016/j.jadohealth.2016.10.020
26. Wyns C, Collienne C, Shenfield F, Robert A, Laurent P, Roegiers L, Brichard B (2015) Fertility preservation in the male pediatric population: factors influencing the decision of parents and children. Hum Reprod 30(9):2022–2030. https://doi.org/10.1093/humrep/dev161
27. Sundberg KK, Lampic C, Arvidson J, Helström L, Wettergren L (2011) Sexual function and experience among long-term survivors of childhood cancer. Eur J Cancer 47(3):397–403. https://doi.org/10.1016/j.ejca.2010.09.040
28. Wettergren L, Kent EE, Mitchell SA, Zebrack B, Lynch CF, Rubenstein MB, THM K, Wu XC, Parsons HM, Smith AW, AYA HOPE Study Collaborative Group (2017) Cancer negatively impacts on sexual function in adolescents and young adults: the AYA HOPE study. Psychooncology 26(10):1632–1639. https://doi.org/10.1002/pon.4181
29. Lehmann V, Gerhardt CA, Baust K, Kaatsch P, Hagedoorn M, Tuinman MA (2022) Psychosexual development and sexual functioning in young adult survivors of childhood cancer. J Sex Med 19(11):1644–1654. https://doi.org/10.1016/j.jsxm.2022.07.014
30. Lehmann V, Hagedoorn M, Gerhardt CA, Fults M, Olshefski RS, Sanderman R, Tuinman MA (2016) Body issues, sexual satisfaction, and relationship status satisfaction in long-term childhood cancer survivors and healthy controls. Psychooncology 25(2):210–216. https://doi.org/10.1002/pon.3841
31. Varela VS, Zhou ES, Bober SL (2013) Management of sexual problems in cancer patients and survivors. Curr Probl Cancer 37:319–352
32. American Psychiatric Association (ed) (2013) Diagnostic and statistical manual of mental disorders, 5th edn. American Psychiatric Association, Washington, DC
33. White ID, Allan H, Faithfull S (2011) Assessment of female sexual morbidity induced by treatment in oncology: is it part of routine medical follow-up after radical pelvic radiotherapy? Br J Cancer 105:903–910

Chapter 4
Male Infertility: From East to West

Male infertility and sexual dysfunctions often coexist and the Asia Pacific Society of Sexual Medicine (APSSM) and the Asian Society of Men's Health and Aging (ASMHA) have provided a series of clinical recommendations based on current evidence to guide physicians in the management of MI (male infertility) and MSD (male sexual dysfunctions) within the Asia-Pacific region (AP).

A thorough review of the published scientific literature (in the MEDLINE and EMBASE databases) was conducted between January 2021 and June 2022 under the keywords: "low libido," "erectile dysfunction," "ejaculatory dysfunction," "premature ejaculation," "retrograde ejaculation," "delayed ejaculation," "anejaculation," and "orgasmic dysfunction."

It is believed that the rate of MI is probably higher in the Asia-Pacific region (AP) compared to Western countries due to locoregional factors such as the uneven distribution of health systems and sociocultural beliefs, especially among patriarchal societies [1]. Prospectively, it is estimated that about a third of the male population will experience at least one form of MSD in their lifetime [2]. The presence of MSD can affect males, negatively impacting on psychosocial functions and interpersonal and relational relationships [3].

In fact, unsuccessful family planning triggers a negative conditioning on the individual's feelings and many couples describe the period of diagnosis and treatment of infertility as the most stressful period of their life [4].

The clinical path of infertility determines the frequency and timing of sexual intercourse; the usually intimate event is regulated, controlled by third parties and often couples sense that the medical team is symbolically present even during their most intimate act [5].

Often problems occur due to the emotional impact of diagnosis and forced sexual intercourse dictated as part of treatment and management of the problem [6].

Studies have shown that both perceived stress and real-life stressful events can be associated with lower sperm quality in the general male population [7].

E. V. Longhi, *Framing Sexual Dysfunctions and Diseases during Fertility Treatment*, https://doi.org/10.1007/978-3-031-76726-5_4

A period of acute psychosocial stress can induce changes in the sexual response up to the point of suppression of testosterone production [8]. It has been found that both sperm quality and testosterone levels appear reduced in infertile men with higher psychological stress compared to infertile men who reported lower stress [9].

4.1 APSSM and ASMHA Consensus Statements

The presence of coexisting MI and MSD induce a dysfunctional sexual response and poor fertility. Similarly to epidemiological data linking MSD to general health, MI can signify a future health problem such as metabolic and hormonal abnormalities that go beyond mere family planning.

Given that MSD are common, and MI seems to be increasing in many parts of the AP region, clinical experience, availability of and access to relevant resources, and the quality of interventions must become relevant to the clinical request. Although there are variations in treatment strategies for managing MI and MSD due to geographical competence, locoregional resources, and sociocultural factors, a comprehensive evaluation of fertility and sexuality with a multidisciplinary management approach is highly recommended. It is important to address the individual issues of male infertility (MI) by emphasizing the improvement of spermatogenesis and facilitating reproductive pathways, while managing various areas of male sexual dysfunction (MSD) with evidence-based treatments. All therapeutic options should be discussed in a shared decision-making process, clinicians and patients, based on contemporary scientific evidence to balance risks, expected outcomes, and available resources. Accompanying the patient and the couple to a reality assessment with more options of probability of success: positive, neutral, null.

4.2 Made in USA

Other American studies (including Berger et al.) have confirmed that male partners of infertile couples experience an increase in sexual stress related to infertility [10], less sexual satisfaction, and worse erectile function; additionally in some specific subtypes of male infertility, the risk of erectile dysfunction significantly increases. Based on these data, existing evidence suggests that male factor infertility can indeed be a risk factor for sexual problems in men.

Although male infertility has been implicated as a risk factor for increased personal distress, no study to date has simultaneously evaluated demographic characteristics, socioeconomic status, racial background, religious affiliation, and fertility history as predictors of the psychosocial impact of male infertility. These elements can significantly contribute to how men perceive the impact of their infertility diagnosis.

It is hypothesized [11] that men in infertile couples who felt responsible for the fertility problem (i.e., with a diagnosis of male factor infertility) would have experienced a greater sexual, marital, social, and personal impact compared to men who did not feel responsible for the couple's infertility.

The study by Smith et al. [11] recruited 380 couples from eight reproductive endocrinology clinics: of these, 357 (94%) male patients completed the survey questionnaires and agreed to individual interviews.

Study participants completed questionnaires at the time of enrollment that contained medical and surgical histories, socioeconomic and demographic data, history of previous paternity, and four psychosocial impact scales: Nancy Adler, PhD; Mary Croughan, PhD; Steven Gregorich, Ph.D.; Susan G. Millstein, PhD; Robert Nachtigall, MD; and Jonathan Showstack, MPH, PhD.

A questionnaire of "Psychosocial Measures Used to Evaluate the Impact of an Infertility Diagnosis," by Smith JF, Walsh TJ, Shindel AW, Turek PJ, Wing H, Pasch L, Katz PP (2009 Sept.) Infertility Outcomes Program Project Group is available at [11].

The average age of the men ($N = 357$) examined was 36.9 years (range 21.7–60, SD 5.5). The average age of the partners was 35.7 years (range 22–46). Non-white men constituted 25% of the sample population, 70% had achieved at least a high school diploma, and 67% had a family income over US$ 100,000 per year.

No male factor (i.e., an isolated female factor) was reported in 47%, the male factor alone was reported in 12%, male and female factors in 16%, and the diagnosis was unexplained in 25%. In contrast to this perceived diagnosis, after a complete evaluation, 58% had only the female factor, 7% had only the male factor, 30% of couples had male and female factors, and only 5% had no known factor. The kappa between the perceived diagnosis at the time of the baseline interview and the actual diagnosis after 18 months was 0.35.

Ultimately, the research results: validated the association between male infertility and dysfunctions in sexual response as well as a lower quality of sperm in patients under stress [12].

Furthermore, male partners of infertile couples may experience worse general mental health as an even greater risk of psychosocial problems and a reduced quality of life.

On average, men with male factor infertility have lower self-esteem and greater feelings of stigmatization and loss of respect from fertile men [13].

Furthermore, patients who are diagnosed with the responsibility for the couple's infertility report lower overall life satisfaction, greater discomfort, and increased treatment-related anxiety after being diagnosed as responsible for the couple's infertility.

The underlying quality of the marriage can influence or predispose men to personal, marital, or sexual tensions; these problems may not be related and precede the diagnosis of infertility.

Marriages with a strong bond can help protect individuals from psychosocial stress factors resulting from a diagnosis of infertility and subsequent treatment [14].

Men with anxiety, depression, or preexisting dysfunctional coping may be more at risk of psychosocial dysfunction in the face of the difficulties of this treatment.

It has been shown that the interaction between stress factors and coping mechanisms within each couple plays a significant role in determining the overall psychosocial impact [15].

It is interesting to note that at the time of enrollment in the study, in couples with male and female factor infertility, men did not experience greater personal, social, sexual, or marital impacts compared to men without male factor infertility.

Couples may have actively supported each other more in this group. It has been shown that spousal support is very important in dealing with the stress resulting from a diagnosis of infertility [16].

A comprehensive study on the coping styles of men and women undergoing in vitro fertilization found that women choose confrontation, acceptance of responsibility and seek social support, and escape/avoidance styles more often than men [15].

They also found that men and women with escape/avoidance mechanisms had the highest levels of infertility-related stress.

4.3 Conclusions

In the diversity of cultures and the ease of access to "specialized centers" for male infertility, each individual requires their own clinical and social history, the development of their own sexuality, cultural, geographical, and political belonging, as well as the role within the couple to be evaluated. These aspects, not traceable from genetics and fertility procedures, are at the basis of the compliance of each patient and each individual couple. Mental well-being, couple relationships, ties with families of origin and social and economic status significantly determine the therapeutic path.

Every clinician, if not prepared in this sense, should be accompanied by a sexologist to build systemic paths to the individual and the couple. Obviously, when the native culture allows it.

References

1. Rutstein SO, Shah IH (2004) Infecundity, infertility and childlessness in developing countries. DHS comparative reports no. 9. ORC Macro, World Health Organization
2. McCabe MP, Sharlip ID, Lewis R, Atalla E, Balon R, Fisher AD et al (2016) Incidence and prevalence of sexual dysfunction in women and men: a consensus statement from the fourth international consultation on sexual medicine. J Sex Med 13:144–152
3. Liu Y, Wang Y, Pu Z, Wang Y, Zhang Y, Dong C et al (2022) Sexual dysfunction in infertile men: a systematic review and meta-analysis. Sex Med 10:100528

4. Piva I, Lo Monte G, Graziano A, Marci R (2014) A literature review on the relationship between infertility and sexual dysfunction: does fun end with making a baby? Eur J Contracept Reprod Health Care 19(4):231–237. https://doi.org/10.3109/13625187.2014.919379
5. Bravermann AM (2004) Psychosocial aspect of infertility: sexual dysfunction. Ser Congr Int 1266:270–276. https://doi.org/10.1016/j.ics.2004.01.085
6. Starc A, Trampuš M, Pavan Jukić D, Rotim C, Jukić T, Polona MA (2019) Infertility and sexual dysfunctions: a systematic literature review. Acta Clin Croat 58(3):508–515. https://doi.org/10.20471/acc.2019.58.03.15
7. Janevic T, Kahn LG, Landsbergis P, Cirillo PM, Cohn BA, Liu X et al (2014) Effects of work and life stress on sperm quality. Fertil Steril 102:530–538
8. Kajantie E, Phillips DI (2006) The effects of sex and hormonal status on the physiological response to acute psychosocial stress. Psychoneuroendocrinology 31:151–178
9. Salvio G, Ciarloni A, Cutini M, Delli Muti N, Finocchi F, Perrone M et al (2022) Metabolic syndrome and male fertility: beyond the cardiac consequences of a complex cardiometabolic endocrinopathy. Int J Mol Sci 23:5497
10. Berger DM (1918) Impotence following the discovery of azoospermia. Fertil Sterile 34:154–156
11. Smith JF, Walsh TJ, Shindel AW, Turek PJ, Wing H, Pasch L, Katz PP, Infertility Outcomes Program Project Group (2009) Sexual, marital, and social impact of a man's perceived infertility diagnosis. J Sex Med 6(9):2505–2515. https://doi.org/10.1111/j.1743-6109.2009.01383.x
12. Eskiocak S, Gozen AS, Kilic AS, Molla S (2005) Association between mental stress and some antioxidant enzymes of seminal plasma. Indian J Med Res 122:491–496
13. Nachtigall RD, Becker G, Wozny M (1992) The effects of gender-specific diagnosis on male and female response to infertility. Fertil Sterile 57:113–121
14. Schneider MG, Forthofer MS (2005) Associations of psychosocial factors with the stress of infertility treatment. Soc Work Health Care 30:183–191
15. Peterson BD, Newton CR, Rosen KH, Skaggs GE (2006) Gender differences in how men and women undergoing in vitro fertilization cope with infertility stress. Hum Reprod 21:2443–2449
16. Daniluk J (1997) Helping patients cope with infertility. Clin Obstet Gynecol 40:661–672

Chapter 5
Eating Disorders, Infertility, Difficult Sexuality

Eating and sexual disorders significantly alter male and female fertility. Obesity, anorexia, bulimia, compulsive behaviors show patients in antagonism with themselves due to body dysmorphia, inadequacy, borderline personality with self-destructive or sabotaging behaviors. Denying the investigation of these factors means evading complex co-causes of infertility and above all, the success of medical procedures. In addition to colluding with therapeutic failures that are easier to avoid and prevent.

First of all, obesity is considered a global health problem that affects about 650 million adults, about 12% of the world population [1]. This pathology increases the risk of associated conditions: type 2 diabetes mellitus, dyslipidemia, cholelithiasis, hypertension, coronary disease, stroke, endometrial and breast cancer, premature aging, and neurodegenerative diseases with a consequent 4,000,000 deaths every year worldwide (equivalent to 7% of global mortality) [2].

Obesity has been associated with reduced fertility: overweight women suffer from alterations of the hypothalamus–pituitary–ovary axis, menstrual cycle disorders, and show a probability up to three times higher of suffering from oligo/anovulation. A delicate hormonal balance regulates follicular development and oocyte maturation. In fact, adipocytes are responsible for the production of a hormone called leptin (present in high quantities in obese women), which has been associated with reduced fertility. In addition, to compromising ovulation, obesity negatively affects the development and implantation of the endometrium. The expression of polycystic ovary syndrome (PCOS) is regulated, in part, by body weight, so obese women with PCOS often have a more severe phenotype and higher rates of subfertility. Finally, obesity compromises women's response to medically assisted procreation (MAP) treatments, as well as influencing fetal, neonatal, and infant development (www.actabiomedica.it) [3].

E. V. Longhi, *Framing Sexual Dysfunctions and Diseases during Fertility Treatment*, https://doi.org/10.1007/978-3-031-76726-5_5

5.1 Obesity and Female Infertility

The World Health Organization (WHO) estimates that about one billion people worldwide are overweight and that over 300 million of them are obese. Obesity seems to derive mainly from the imbalance between reduced physical exercise, excessive intake of high-calorie foods, changes in lifestyle, and diet composition. In 2013, the American Medical Association recognized obesity as a systemic disease. Most obese women are not sterile; however, obesity and its negative impact on fecundity and fertility are well documented. Research results have shown that obesity damages fertility through its negative effects on the control of ovulation, the development of oocytes, embryos, and the endometrium, as well as compromising the progression and overall quality of implantation. Obese women are three times more likely to suffer from infertility compared to women with a normal BMI [4].

Marinelli et al. [5] conducted an in-depth study on the impact of obesity on female fertility, evaluating research collected in PubMed/Medline, Embase, Web of Science, drawing on sources covering the period 1994–2022. One hundred and twenty-four sources were identified in addition to considering the guidelines and recommendations of the International Federation of Gynecology and Obstetrics, the American Society of Reproductive Medicine, the British Fertility Society, the Canadian Task Force on Preventive Health Care, the American Association of Clinical Endocrinologists (AACE), and the American College of Endocrinology including also patients undergoing assisted reproduction techniques.

The results are as follows:

1. Obese women may have reduced fertility mainly due to a lower frequency of sexual intercourse, despite the presence of cohabiting partners, and to excess fats and sugars in the diet, responsible for the attenuation of libido [6].
2. The distribution of body fat would also have significant repercussions on the reproductive abilities of couples and it has been observed that central obesity, defined by an increase in waist circumference or by a high WHR (waist–hip ratio), has a negative impact on fertility. A Dutch study showed that an increase of 0.1 units of WHR is correlated with a 30% decrease in the probability of conception per cycle [7]. Obesity can produce effects on the hypothalamus–pituitary–ovary (HPO) axis and, in fact, severely obese women show a rate of menstrual disorders 3.1 times higher than normal weight women [8].
3. But that is not all. These patients show high rates of spontaneous abortion both after natural conception and after MAP programs, which is a significantly higher probability of experiencing a spontaneous abortion, regardless of the mode of conception [9].
4. A retrospective analysis of women with PCOS undergoing ovulation induction showed a higher abortion rate among obese women (BMI > 28 kg/m^2) compared to the normal weight female population (60% vs. 27%). The analysis of 5019 IVF/ICSI cycles in 2660 women in a Norwegian clinic observed an index of early spontaneous abortion (<6 weeks) or miscarriage (6–12 weeks). The OR for

early pregnancy termination was 1.69 (95% CI 1.13–2.51, $P = 0.003$) in obese women (BMI > 30 kg/m^2) compared to normal weight women.

Furthermore, an incorrect diet from childhood would have a negative impact on the intestine and on the composition of the microbiome, leading to obesity and possibly to colorectal cancer (CRC) in adults [10]. Other authors, on the other hand, have reported an increase in spontaneous abortion rates, attributing this condition to a reduction in oocyte quality or to an alteration in embryonic development [11]. A reduced ability to develop the oocyte can compromise the potential development of the embryo, which can lead to an implantation/invasion anomaly of the trophoblast.

Poor reproductive prospects in obese women, both in natural and assisted conception cycles, may be the result of a combination of lower implantation rates, higher indices of preclinical and clinical abortions, and greater pregnancy complications for both the mother and the fetus. It is known that obesity causes hormonal changes that have important effects on endometrial function, embryo implantation, and abnormal proliferation, which can also lead to endometrial hyperplasia [12].

A study involving 20 women undergoing in vitro fertilization found that weight fluctuations affect the success of the treatment: an increase in BMI unit significantly reduces the likelihood of achieving a pregnancy (after in vitro fertilization) by 0.84 and, conversely, weight loss improves the chances of achieving a pregnancy by a factor of 1.19 per unit [13].

The British Fertility Society has stated that obese patients should aim to lower their body mass index to normal levels before undertaking any form of ART procedure [14]. Any fertility treatment should be postponed until the patient's BMI is below 35 kg/m^2, although in patients under 37 years (therefore with more fertile years available) with a normal serum concentration of FSH, it would be advisable to aim for an even lower BMI (below 30 kg/m^2).

Regarding chronological age: In Europe, 34 out of 43 countries have legal age limits for the treatment of couple infertility and the Czech Republic, Denmark, Greece, Portugal, Spain, Sweden, and the United Kingdom set the age for men and women to access assisted fertilization techniques at 18 years. The maximum female age is also a legal limit in 18 countries, ranging from 45 years in Denmark and Belgium (in the latter this limit applies to egg retrieval while embryo replacement and insemination are allowed up to 47 years) to 51 in Bulgaria. There are no legal age limits in Finland, Germany, Norway, while the current legislation in Spain sets a maximum limit for women at the age of "menopause" and in the Netherlands at the age of 49 years. Some countries, including Austria, Hungary, and Poland, have not set an age limit to grant access to MAP. The Italian Constitutional Court, in the judgments that have modified law no. 40 of 2004 [15], has clearly stated that the legislator cannot impose decisions on technical-scientific issues, but must allow experts or doctors to reasonably adapt the rules to different situations.

It is therefore up to the doctor to determine what risks an obese woman would run following the application of a technique (e.g., ovarian stimulation), achieving pregnancy (probability of miscarriage, for example) or childbirth, following a thorough clinical examination evaluation on a case-by-case basis and considering the general conditions of the patient.

5.2 The Influence of Body Image

Considering all these factors, female sexual response and fertility are also determined by the "body image," that is to say intrapsychic, social factors, beyond marital satisfaction, relationship stability, and communication [16].

What is this about?

Women's body image is conditioned by specific parts of the body that they would like to be different (flatter abdomen, muscular arms, and thighs), body weight, height, comparison with their own body in front of a partner or other women [17].

An extreme manifestation of body dissatisfaction is often reported by patients with eating disorders in which the distorted body image leads to pathological eating behaviors [18].

In fact, the eating behavior of infertile women seems to be more disturbed compared to the general population [19, 20].

The prevalence of eating disorders has been estimated to be between 8% and 16% (including obesity, anorexia, and bulimia) among infertile women with a progression of the phenomenon up to 44% if past phenomena (childhood, adolescence) or following sexual abuse are taken into account [21].

Consequently, the evaluation of the desire for a child must take into account body satisfaction, eating, and sexual dysfunctions, as well as the causes of infertility.

Patients with eating disorders show endocrine alterations, functional amenorrhea before a significant loss (20–25%) of weight [22], during dieting (50–75%), low self-esteem, couple problems, and hormonal therapy intake.

A study on 151 patients with a history of eating disorders and a desire for motherhood showed (even 13 years after hospital contact) that the desire for a child was ambivalent or only fantasized [23].

Research questionnaires help a lot to explore some characteristics of future parents:

1. The questionnaire FKW (Frageboden zum Kinderwunsch) identifies expectations and apprehensions related to motherhood, birth, and parenthood using 20 evaluation questions (1 = not at all to 5 = very true) [24]. Three hypotheses were evaluated: improvement of self-esteem, emotional stability, ambivalence in the relationship.
2. The BSQ (Body Shape Questionnaire) evaluates the concerns about weight and shape: a score above 140 indicates a very intense concern. Hence, social avoidance and shame in showing one's body, body dissatisfaction especially from the waist down, use of laxatives and vomiting to reduce body dissatisfaction, obsessiveness in weight control [25].

3. The Hospital Anxiety and Depression Scale (HAD) evaluates anxiety (HAD-A) and depression (HAD-D) based on 14 items. A score of 7 or less indicates a "normal" level, between 8 and 10 a "borderline" level, and 11 or more a "pathological" level of anxiety and depression.
4. The FertiQoL measures the quality of life in infertile patients. It consists of 24 items that evaluate the emotional aspects, the mind/body relationship, the relational and social aspect, and physical health [26].

5.3 Management of Obesity Prepregnancy, during Pregnancy, Postpartum

Guidelines from the FIGO Committee for the management of prepregnancy obesity, pregnancy, and postpartum examine the recommendations of good clinical practice from previously published international documents. It serves as a practical resource to support obstetricians and gynecologists in the management of women with obesity.

Time point A: Prepregnancy	
A.1	All women should have their weight and height measured and their body mass index (BMI; calculated as weight in kilograms divided by height in meters squared) calculated. Consider ethnic differences.
A.2	All women with a BMI of ≥30 should be advised of the effect of obesity on fertility, the immediate risks of obesity during pregnancy and childbirth, and the subsequent long-term health effect of obesity including the higher risk of noncommunicable diseases for them and their children.
A.3	All women with obesity should be encouraged to lose weight through diet and adopting a healthy lifestyle including moderate physical activity. If indicated and available, other weight management interventions might be considered, including bariatric surgery.
A.4	All women with obesity should be advised to take at least 0.4 mg (400 μg) and consider up to 5 mg folic acid supplementation daily for at least 1–3 months before conception.
Time point B: Pregnancy	
B.1	All women should have their weight and height measured and their BMI calculated at the first antenatal visit. Consider ethnic differences. Advise on appropriate gestational weight gain.
B.2	All women should receive information on diet and lifestyle appropriate to their gestation including nutrient supplements, weight management, and regular physical activity.
B.3	All women with obesity should be advised of the risks of obesity and excess gestational weight gain on pregnancy, childbirth, and long-term health including risk of noncommunicable diseases for them and their children.
B.4	All antenatal healthcare facilities should have well-defined multidisciplinary pathways for the clinical management of pregnant women with obesity including the identification and treatment of pregnancy-related complications.
Time point C: Postpartum	
C.1	All women with prepregnancy obesity should receive support on breastfeeding initiation and maintenance.

C.2	All women with obesity and pregnancy complications should receive appropriate postnatal follow-up in line with local resources, care pathways, and in response to the individual health requirements of each woman and her children.
C.3	All women with obesity should be encouraged to lose weight postpartum with emphasis on healthy diet, breastfeeding if possible, and regular moderate physical activity. They should be advised of the importance of long-term follow-up as they and their children are at increased risk for noncommunicable diseases.
C.4	Maternal obesity should be considered when making the decision regarding the most appropriate form of postnatal contraception.

It is hypothesized that by 2025 more than 21% of women will suffer from obesity worldwide [28]. In the United States, the NHANES (National Health and Nutrition Examination Survey) 2011–2012 data indicate that the prevalence of obesity in women aged between 20 and 39 years is at least 31.8% and seems to be even higher in low-income women at 61% [29].

The prevalence of maternal obesity varies in different African nations, ranging from 17.9% in the first trimester to 6.5–50.7% in the third trimester [30].

In many countries, routine surveillance of weight gain during pregnancy does not seem to be conducted. However, the body mass index (BMI) among women of reproductive age is often used as an indicator of maternal obesity and its likely effect on pregnancy outcomes and the subsequent health of the woman and child.

Global clinical experience shows that obese women are more likely to have nutritional deficiencies (e.g., of vitamin D, iron, and vitamin B12) compared to women with a lower BMI [31].

Furthermore, women with a BMI ≥ 30 would have a higher risk of anxiety and depression.

But worse, some scientific studies have linked infertility, obesity, pre- and postpartum depression with child abuse.

The study by Nagl et al. [32] examined 741 women at 16 weeks postpartum ($M = 8.1$ weeks, SD = 3.2). Child sexual, physical, and emotional abuse and physical and emotional neglect were assessed with the Childhood Trauma Questionnaire. Depression and anxiety were assessed using BDI and SCL-90-R.

Results: 7.6% of the included women entered pregnancy with obesity. 46% reported some type of child abuse. 6.4% showed at least moderate postnatal depressive symptoms and 20.5% scored above the 75th percentile for postpartum anxiety. Severe physical abuse, moderate emotional abuse, and severe physical and emotional neglect were associated with prepregnancy obesity. After controlling for the presence of all other types of child abuse, only severe physical abuse was still predictive of prepregnancy obesity (OR adj. = 5.24, 95% CI = 1.15–23.75). Prepregnancy obesity was associated with an increased risk of postpartum depression (OR adj. = 2.55, 95% CI = 1.08–6.00), but not with high anxiety. Prepregnancy obesity and severe child sexual abuse independently predicted postpartum depression.

It was found that child abuse is associated with both prepregnancy obesity and the impairment of postpartum mental health and can at least partly explain the association between prepregnancy obesity and postpartum depression. Therefore, child maltreatment is related to two common risk conditions during pregnancy and postpartum that involve various risks to the health of the mother and child.

5.4 Conclusions

The scientific literature shows how sexual dysfunctions and eating disorders are present in infertile couples, even in their past history. Moreover, infertile patients often show mood or personality disorders compared to fertile women [27]. Couples seek a child at all costs and their desire is often conditioned by a reserved quality of life, scarcely social, and symbiotic. The ambivalence between the desire and the real choice to undertake a fertilization process seems more a consequence of the lack of planning by the couple than an objective search. Anxiety and depressive behaviors, more present in subjects with eating disorders, are exacerbated with the prolongation of medical therapies.

Thus, self-esteem and the couple's relationship show inadequacy, dissatisfaction, lack of sociocultural stimuli, invasiveness of families of origin. Lastly, the specialists are more attentive to the feasibility of fertilization procedures than these aspects. The sexologist is a figure sometimes confused with the psychologist or psychiatrist.

The teams question themselves "if," "when," "with which couples" to propose a sexological screening a priori to assess the quality of the couple's relationship.

The desire for a child often appears associated with a degrading sexuality, which is barely gratifying and repetitive. So much so that they see in the newborn the magical solution to negate the problem.

There is still much to do to give the right sense to the history of couples and not just to the desire for parenthood. Perhaps many frustrations and failures can be avoided.

References

1. Afshin A, at all. (2017) Health effects of overweight and obesity in 195 countries over 25 years. N Engl Med 377(1):13–27
2. Kelly T, Yang W, Chen CS, Reynolds K, He J (2008) Global burden of obesity in 2005 and projections to 2030. Int J Obesity 32(9):1431–1437
3. Rich-Edwards JW, Goldman MB, Willett WC, Hunter DJ, Stampfer MJ, Colditz GA, Manson JE (1994) Adolescent body mass index and infertility caused by ovulatory disorder. Am J Obstet Gynecol 171(1):171–177. https://doi.org/10.1016/0002-9378(94)90465-0
4. Bezerra Espinola MS, Laganà AS, Bilotta G, Gullo G, Aragona C, Unfer V (2021) D-chiro-inositol induces ovulation in non-polycystic ovary syndrome (PCOS), young non-insulin resistant women, probably modulating aromatase expression: a report of 2 cases. Am J Case Rep 22:e932722

5. Marinelli S, Napoletano G, Straccamore M, Basile G (2022) Female obesity and infertility: outcomes and regulatory guidance. Acta Biomed 93(4):e2022278. https://doi.org/10.23750/abm.v93i4.13466
6. Hassan MA, Killick SR (2004) A negative lifestyle is associated with a significant reduction in fertility. Fertil Sterile 81:384–392
7. Zaadstra BM, Seidell JC, Van Noord PA et al (1993) Fat and female fertility: prospective study of the effect of body fat distribution on conception rates. BMJ 306:484–487
8. Gesink Law DC, Maclehose RF, Longnecker MP (2007) Obesity and time to pregnancy. Hum Reprod 22:414–420
9. Metwally M, Ong KJ, Ledger WL, Li TC (2008) Does a high body mass index increase the risk of miscarriage after spontaneous and assisted conception? A meta-analysis of the evidence. Fertil Steril 90:714–726
10. Campisciano G, de Manzini N, Delbue S, Cason C, Cosola D, Basile G, Ferrante P, Comar M, Palmisano S (2020) The obesity-related gut bacterial and viral dysbiosis can impact the risk of colon cancer development. Microorganisms 8(3):431. https://doi.org/10.3390/microorganisms8030431
11. Chen R, Chen L, Liu Y, Wang F, Wang S, Huang Y, Hu KL, Fan Y, Liu R, Zhang R, Zhang D (2021) Association of parental prepregnancy BMI with neonatal outcomes and birth defect in fresh embryo transfer cycles: a retrospective cohort study. BMC Pregnancy Childbirth 21(1):793. https://doi.org/10.1186/s12884-021-04261-y
12. Bellver J, Marín C, Lathi RB, Murugappan G, Labarta E, Vidal C, Giles J, Cabanillas S, Marzal A, Galliano D, Ruiz-Alonso M, Simón C, Valbuena D (2021) Obesity affects endometrial receptivity by shifting the implantation window. Reprod Sci 28:3171–3180
13. Fridström M, Sjöblom P, Pousette A, Hillensjö T (1997) Serum FSH levels in women with polycystic ovary syndrome during ovulation induction using down-regulation and urofollitropin. Eur J Endocrinol 136(5):488–492. https://doi.org/10.1530/eje.0.1360488
14. Bellver J, Busso C, Pellicer A, Remohi J, Simon C (2006) Obesity and outcomes of assisted reproduction technology. Reprod Biomed Online 12:562–568
15. Bhakuni H, Miotto L (2021) Conscientious objection to abortion in the developing world: the argument of correspondence. Dev World Bioeth 21:90–95
16. Waite LJ, Joyner K (2001) Emotional satisfaction and physical pleasure in sexual unions: Time horizon, sexual behavior, and sexual exclusivity. J Marriage Fam 63(1):247–264. https://doi.org/10.1111/j.1741-3737.2001.00247.x
17. Wiedermann M (2000) Women's self-awareness of body image during sexual intimacy with a partner. J Sex Res 37:60–68
18. Stice E (2002) Risk and maintenance factors for eating pathology: a meta-analytic review. Psychol Bull 128:825–848
19. Lamas C, Nicolas I, Alvarez L, Hoffmann M, Buisson G, Gérardin P (2014) Problems of maternal eating behavior during the perinatal period: a problem of prevention of early development and parenting problems. EMC Psychiatry. VII:37–54
20. Stewart DE, Robinson E, Goldbloom DS, Wright C (1990) Infertility and eating disorders. Am J Obstet Gynecol 163(4 Pt 1):1196–1199. https://doi.org/10.1016/0002-9378(90)90688-4
21. Freizinger M, Franko DL, Dacey M, Okun B, Domar AD (2010) The prevalence of eating disorders in infertile women. Fertil Steril 93(1):72–78. https://doi.org/10.1016/j.fertnstert.2008.09.055
22. Mehler PS, Brown C (2015) Anorexia nervosa—medical complications. J Eat Disord 3:11. https://doi.org/10.1186/s40337-015-0040-8
23. Brinch M, Isager T, Tolstrup K (1988) Anorexia nervosa and motherhood: reproduction pattern and mothering behavior of 50 women. Acta Psychiatr Scand 77(5):611–617. https://doi.org/10.1111/j.1600-0447.1988.tb05175.x
24. Hölzle C, Wirtz M (2001) Fragebogen zum Kinderwunsch: FKW; Manual. Hogrefe, Verlag für Psychologie, Göttingen, p 110

25. Rousseau A, Knotter A, Barbe P, Raich R, Chabrol H (2005) Etude de validation de la version française du Body Shape Questionnaire [Validation of the French version of the Body Shape Questionnaire]. Encéphale 31(2):162–173. French. https://doi.org/10.1016/s0013-7006(05)82383-8
26. Boivin J, Takefman J, Braverman A (2011) The fertility quality of life (FertiQoL) tool: development and general psychometric properties. Hum Reprod 26(8):2084–2091. https://doi.org/10.1093/humrep/der171
27. Sbaragli C, Morgante G, Goracci A, Hofkens T, De Leo V, Castrogiovanni P (2008) Infertility and psychiatric morbidity. Fertil Steril 90(6):2107–2111. https://doi.org/10.1016/j.fertnstert.2007.10.045
28. Zhou B, Lu Y, Hajifathalian K, Bentham J, Di Cesare M, Danaei G, Bixby H, Cowan MJ, Ali MK, Taddei C, Lo WC (2016) Worldwide trends in diabetes since 1980: a pooled analysis of 751 population-based studies with 4· 4 million participants. Lancet 387(10027):1513–1530
29. Ogden CL, Carroll MD, Kit BK, Flegal KM (2014) Prevalence of childhood and adult obesity in the United States, 2011–2012. JAMA 311:806–814
30. Onubi OJ, Marais D, Aucott L, Okonofua F, Poobalan AS (2016) Maternal obesity in Africa: a systematic review and a meta-analysis. J Public Health 38:e218–e231
31. Denison FC, Aedla NR, Keag O, Hor K, Reynolds RM, Milne A, Diamond A, on behalf of the Royal College of Obstetricians and Gynaecologists (2019) Care of women with obesity in pregnancy. BJOG 126:e62–e106
32. Nagl M, Lehnig F, Stepan H, Wagner B, Kersting A (2017) Associations of childhood maltreatment with pre-pregnancy obesity and maternal postpartum mental health: a cross-sectional study. BMC Pregnancy Childbirth 17(1):391

Chapter 6
Infertility and COVID-19

In recent years, significant progress has been made in understanding the link between COVID-19 infection and male infertility. Although the data is still limited, there is enough information available to draw some conclusions [1].

Immediately after infection, sperm quality appears to be suppressed through mechanisms that seem to lower testosterone levels and alter all aspects of the sperm profile (sperm count, motility, and morphology, as well as leukocyte infiltration). The extent of the effect depends on the severity and duration of the disease [2].

It seems that damage to sperm DNA is a feature of the disease that could have an impact not only on the fertility of affected patients but also on the health and well-being of their offspring [3]. It is hypothesized that these effects on sperm quality decrease over time, although further studies are needed to prove this point. It is not yet clear whether changes in sperm quality reflect a direct impact of the virus on spermatogenesis and sperm function or whether it is an indirect reflection of the cytokine storm triggered by the disease and the consequent increase in oxidative stress.

A careful application of antioxidants in combination with oxidative stress biomarkers to monitor the effectiveness of the latter would constitute a rational approach toward solving this problem, as suggested by Marin et al. [3]. In the last 12 months, significant progress has been made in understanding the link between COVID-19 infection and male infertility. Enough information is available to draw some general conclusions and suggest future research paths.

Although complete data is lacking, a growing number of studies suggest that testicular endocrine function, i.e., the secretion of testosterone, was compromised during acute COVID-19 infection [4], and more severe disease is associated with lower testosterone levels [5].

It is not known whether these men had lower testosterone levels before SARS-CoV-2 infection or whether the virus affects androgen production. Studies have been conducted suggesting the latter hypothesis, as they have shown that testosterone levels were low during infection but increased during the recovery phase, at

E. V. Longhi, *Framing Sexual Dysfunctions and Diseases during Fertility Treatment*, https://doi.org/10.1007/978-3-031-76726-5_6

least in a percentage of men infected with COVID-19 [6]. However, hypogonadism, defined by a decrease in testosterone levels, was observed in about half of the patients during and after recovery from COVID-19 (in studies with a follow-up from 71 days to 7 months) [7].

On the other hand, some authors do not report differences in sperm morphology between mild and moderate disease [8], whereas other publications support the evidence of a strong correlation between sperm parameters and disease severity [9]. It seems, however, that the infection affects spermatogenesis and that this effect can last at least for an entire spermatogenic cycle after recovery.

It remains to be clarified whether the impairment of spermatogenesis is due to direct or indirect effects of the infection. Specific pathogenic mechanisms of the virus, including viral replication and spread leading to inflammation and testicular damage, along with the effect of fever, drugs, and psychological stress due to COVID-19, may play complementary roles. In addition, the immune response in testicular tissues and in the epididymis during SARS-CoV-2 infection could involve an impairment of spermatogenesis [10].

In the study by Rambhatla et al. [11], 32 men diagnosed with COVID-19 who were on replacement therapy with testosterone were compared with 63 men with COVID-19 but not on testosterone treatment. It is interesting to note that no association was found between testosterone treatment and the outcome of COVID-19 in terms of hospital admission, admission to the intensive care unit, further complications, or death.

6.1 COVID-19: Impact on Ovarian Reserve and Follicular Function

Alterations in ovarian reserve and sex hormone-related function could result from a viral infection, such as SARS-CoV-2, and have a potential impact on fertility and fecundity. Studies have evaluated the levels of anti-Müllerian hormone (AMH), antral follicle count (AFC), follicle-stimulating hormone (FSH), luteinizing hormone (LH), estradiol, prolactin, and testosterone in women with COVID-19. Early follicular phase serum levels of FSH, LH, estradiol, and AMH were similar between women hospitalized for COVID-19 and control groups [12]. Similarly, the difference between AMH levels measured within 12 months before and those measured at the start of an ART cycle was similar in asymptomatic women who tested positive or negative for COVID-19 at the start of the ART cycle [13].

Conversely, significantly lower serum AMH levels were reported in 78 women with COVID-19 compared to 151 age-matched healthy controls [14]. This study also reported higher levels of FSH, prolactin, and testosterone in patients with COVID-19. This suggests pituitary and ovarian dysfunction associated with a viral infection, but the validity of this conclusion remains to be confirmed as the study results may have been influenced by a difference in the timing of sample collection (i.e., different phase of the menstrual cycle) between patients and controls.

Regarding ovarian function, a small study compared IgG positive patients from previous cases of COVID-19 with a control group, all undergoing ovarian stimulation for ART [15]. Result? The serum level of estradiol (on the day of ovulation trigger), the estradiol/oocyte ratio, serum progesterone levels on the day of oocyte retrieval, concentrations of estradiol and progesterone in the follicular fluid, the oocyte/aspirated follicles ratio, and the rates of oocyte maturation were similar between the groups. An observational study that evaluated ovarian parameters in 132 women with unexplained infertility before and after COVID-19 reported no statistically significant differences in terms of serum levels of AMH, FSH, LH, FSH/LH ratio, or estradiol levels [16]. Nine months had passed between the two evaluations.

A small study by Morris [17] questioned whether the presence of the SARS-CoV-2 S protein affected the outcome of ART treatments. Consequently, the researchers compared the results of frozen ET in women seropositive to the SARS-CoV-2 vaccine, seropositive to infection, and seronegative: the result was that both implantation rates and clinical pregnancy rates were similar between the groups.

Similarly, immune patients (recovered from COVID-19 infection or who had received the SARS-CoV-2 mRNA vaccine) were compared with patients considered nonimmune and with those treated before the pandemic. Here too, the implantation rates and rates of clinical pregnancy results were comparable [18]. In conclusion, it should be noted that since the beginning of the pandemic, the ESHRE (European Society of Human Reproduction and Embryology) [19], such as other professional societies has recommended a cautious approach to assisted reproduction to avoid further stress to overloaded health systems, but also based on the uncertainty about the effect of the SARS-CoV-2 virus on reproduction and on pregnancy. However, research has continued through the studies of Lambalk et al. [20] and Veiga et al. [21].

6.2 COVID-19 Vaccines and Fertility

AND AGAIN: Is There an Impact of COVID-19 Vaccines on Fertility of Men and Women of Reproductive Age?

Up to June 8, 2022, suitable studies were collected in the databases PubMed, Scopus, Web of Science, Cochrane, and Embase. The quality of the studies was evaluated using the scales Newcastle-Ottawa and Before and After Quality Assessment, respectively, for cohort and pre–post studies [22].

During the first year of the spread of severe acute respiratory syndrome coronavirus-2 (SARS-CoV-2) infection, the only measures available to counter it were personal distancing, the use of protective masks, early identification and isolation of positive patients and their family members. Subsequently, starting from December 2020, vaccines began to be available as the main tool to fight the pandemic [23].

The European Medicines Agency (EMA) and the Food and Drug Administration (FDA) [24] have issued emergency authorization [25] for COVID-19 vaccines, although some subjects have requested their suspension, arguing that the vaccines caused irreparable damage to health and the general population and carried the risk of female infertility [26].

It was hypothesized that the possible mechanism that presumably linked vaccines to the impairment of fertility in women in reproductive age was cross-reactivity with syncytin-1, suggesting a similarity between it and the spike protein. Syncytin-1 plays an essential role in implantation and its dysfunction could indicate a failed implantation, an early pregnancy loss or subsequent problems related to abnormal placentation such as preeclampsia. In males, it was assumed that the vaccine could affect spermatogenesis and sperm parameters, considering that the SARS-CoV-2 virus has been associated with an impairment of male fertility [27].

Returning to the review of the scientific literature by Zaçe et al. [22], it emerged that of the 1406 studies examined, 29 were included in the systematic review. These studies, conducted in Israel (34.5%), the United States (24.1%), Russia (20.7%), China (10.3%), Italy (3.5%), North America (3.5%), and Turkey (3.5%) concerned the poorer classes (34.5%), the upper-middle class (58.6%), and upper class (6.9%). Meta-analyses were performed for progressive sperm motility, pre- and postvaccination, and for concentration. The rate of biochemical and clinical pregnancy did not differ between the vaccinated and unvaccinated groups.

The study by Aharon et al. [28] also seems to follow the same line. The research included patients undergoing controlled ovarian hyperstimulation or transfer of thawed–refrozen euploid embryos. The cycles of controlled ovarian hyperstimulation and the cycles of transfer of thawed–refrozen embryos were evaluated separately. The study groups for controlled ovarian hyperstimulation and the cohorts for transfer of thawed–refrozen embryos consisted of fully vaccinated patients, defined as patients who had received two doses of the Pfizer-BioNTech (Pfizer) or Moderna COVID-19 vaccine. The control groups consisted of unvaccinated patients undergoing controlled ovarian hyperstimulation or transfer of thawed and refrozen embryos during the same time period. Patients who started the drug cycle less than 14 days after the second dose of an mRNA vaccine or who received the Johnson & Johnson/Janssen vaccine in a single solution were excluded from the study.

The patients investigated had taken the first and second dose from February to September 2021. In addition, screening for SARS-CoV-2 infection was performed before each patient visit and procedure and included symptom questionnaires, temperature checks, and vaccination status once vaccines became available. Proof of vaccination, the type and dates of vaccination were entered into the medical record. Tests for SARS-CoV-2 infection were not routinely performed.

A total of 1678 patients undergoing controlled ovarian hyperstimulation and 1271 undergoing single euploid thawed–refrozen embryo transfers were identified. Monthly vaccination rates ranged from 2.7% in February 2021 to 30.7% in May 2021 and were slightly higher in the thawed–refrozen embryo transfer cohort compared to the controlled ovarian hyperstimulation cohort. The controlled ovarian hyperstimulation cohort included 222 fully vaccinated patients and 983 unvaccinated patients. The control group had a higher parity than the vaccinated group. The vaccinated group had a higher percentage of antagonists.

Results: The primary outcome of the fertilization rate for the controlled ovarian hyperstimulation cohort was similar between the vaccinated and unvaccinated groups (80.7% vs. 78.7%). No differences were observed between vaccinated and unvaccinated patients in the univariate analysis of secondary outcomes of eggs retrieved, mature oocytes retrieved, mature oocyte ratio, or blastulation rate. In cycles where preimplantation genetic testing for aneuploidy was performed, vaccinated patients had a higher percentage of euploid embryos compared to unvaccinated patients. The results of this study are also consistent with studies conducted so far on in vitro fertilization outcomes in vaccinated patients.

It is therefore concluded that the administration of mRNA vaccines for COVID-19 was not associated with the development of oocytes or embryos, implantation, or early miscarriage in patients undergoing in vitro fertilization [10]. These results provide further reassuring data that COVID-19 vaccination does not negatively impact fertility or early pregnancy outcomes and contribute to the growing body of evidence that the risk–benefit ratio supports vaccination in pregnant women or those seeking to conceive.

Another proof of this hypothesis is corroborated by the study of Applebaum et al. [29]. Patients undergoing cycles of fresh or frozen embryo transfer at an academic center between January 1, 2020 and December 31, 2021 with a two-dose regimen (Pfizer or Moderna) or a one-dose regimen (Johnson & Johnson/Janssen) before the start of the fertility cycle were evaluated.

Results: Among 709 cycles with unvaccinated patients and 648 cycles of vaccinated women, no statistically significant differences were observed between the number of oocytes retrieved, the maturity of the oocytes, fertilization, and blastocyst utilization rates. Among the 264 cycles of frozen embryo transfer (FET) in unvaccinated and 423 in vaccinated patients, vaccinated patients had higher chances of clinical pregnancy and live births per embryo transfer compared to unvaccinated patients.

6.3 Pandemic, Infertility, and Suspension of Treatments

That being said, we must consider that both infertility and the coronavirus pandemic have had negative mental outcomes, so if the impact of treatment suspension is added, the severity of adverse effects on mental health in infertile patients would significantly increase.

Infertile patients facing suspension or postponement of treatment may be at higher risk of mental disorders. Consequently, the mental health status of an infertile patient undergoing fertility treatment could be different from that of a patient who has had a treatment delay. This difference can affect the quality of life and treatment satisfaction. The team of Dellazizzo et al. [30] conducted a systematic review to assess the mental health of infertile patients facing treatment suspension due to the Covid-19 pandemic.

To conduct this study, the MOOSE guidelines for meta-analyses and systematic reviews of observational studies [31] were followed. The protocol is registered in PROSPERO (International Prospective Register of Systematic Reviews) with the code CRD42023399725. Moreover, the study was approved by the Local Research Ethics Committee, Mashhad University of Medical Sciences, Mashhad, Iran.

A search was conducted through the library databases PubMed, Web of Science, Scopus, PsycINFO, Embase, and Cochrane using keywords including coronavirus, COVID-19, SARS-CoV-2, infertility, assisted reproduction technique, psychological distress, stress, anxiety, depression, psychological state, psychological problems/issues, mental health, suspension, and postponement with no time limits until December 31, 2022. Six hundred and eighty-one studies were identified and 269 studies were screened for inclusion criteria, while 242 studies were excluded [32–35].

Seven studies came from Europe (France [15], Italy [16], Portugal [17], Serbia [18], and Spain [19]); four studies came from Asia (China [20] and India [21]); another four studies came from the Middle East (Iran [22], Israel [23], and Turkey [24]); and six studies were conducted in Canada and/or the United States [25–27]. All participants ($n = 5901$) were infertile patients seeking care during the COVID-19 pandemic and their treatment plans were interrupted or postponed; the majority were women (90%, $n = 5306$), and 8.5% ($n = 504$) of the participants were male. Furthermore, 91 participants (1.5%) did not mention their own gender.

To measure the anxiety of infertile patients, the following were used: Depression, Anxiety, and Stress Scale-21 (DASS-21). Two studies have reported an increase in the anxiety rate in patients who were in isolation [28, 29]. It was reported that the fear of COVID-19 infection and exposure to COVID-19-related news had a negative effect on patients' anxiety [36], especially in women. Furthermore, 64.4% of infertile patients wanted to resume treatment despite the ongoing COVID-19 pandemic. Only 6% of infertile patients agreed to delay treatment and only 28% of infertile patients were worried about mother-to-fetus transmission of the virus in the case of infection during treatment [37]. In the Netherlands (as in the Arab Emirates), due to the COVID-19 pandemic, much elective healthcare such as reproductive medicine was suspended [38–41].

Upon the resumption of healthcare, *video consultation* was used as a new solution to continue consultations in line with the new government rules of social distancing [32]. The fertility workup consisted of two separate video consultations, with diagnostic tests according to a protocol. After the last video consultation, couples received a digital questionnaire, which consisted of a modified version of the Patient-Centered Questionnaire-Infertility (PCQ-I) and the CollaboRATE questionnaire. Fifty-three eligible infertile couples were contacted and of these 22 participated. Four women were contacted for a semi-structured interview [42–45].

Patients mentioned privacy, reduced travel times, and the ease of use of the program as possible advantages of video consultation. However, patients preferred that the first consultation with their doctor took place in person as the video consultation was considered less personal.

Regarding doctors, are there differences in the attitudes and perceptions of doctors toward video and audio consultations during the provision of telemedicine services during the COVID-19 pandemic? [39, 46–49].

The study by Alhajri et al. [50] was conducted on a group of 880 doctors from outpatient facilities in Abu Dhabi, who provided telemedicine services during the COVID-19 pandemic between November and December 2020. In total, 623 doctors responded. The survey included a 5-point Likert scale to measure the attitudes and perceptions of the doctor toward video and audio consultations with reference to the quality of the clinical consultation and professional productivity. Descriptive statistics were used to outline the sociodemographic characteristics of the doctors (age, sex, designation, clinical specialty, duration of practice, and previous experience with telemedicine) and the mode of telemedicine (video vs. audio consultations).

Compared to audio consultations, video consultations were significantly associated with doctors' confidence in managing acute consultations and a greater ability to provide patient education during the web consultation. No significant difference was found in doctors' confidence in managing long-term and follow-up consultations through video or audio consultations. Video consultations were less likely to be associated with a reduction in the overall consultation time and a reduction in the time for the patient to take notes compared to in-person visits.

6.4 Conclusions

Him, Her, and Psychological Experiences During COVID-19

Speaking more closely about the infertile couple and their feelings during COVID-19, Dube et al. [51] conducted an online survey of patients and healthcare workers about their experiences, particularly those of the patients. Five themes emerged: (1) anxiety, (2) mood disorders, (3) threat to self-esteem, identity, and purpose, (4) deterioration of the couple, and (5) weakened support network.

In particular, women reported anxiously thinking about their infertility, often to the point of becoming "obsessed." The inability to access centers dedicated to infertility treatment instilled in couples a sense of absolute powerlessness and loneliness. The parenting process was often experienced as an uphill journey with no possible solution. This lack of participation and control over therapies, mostly interrupted due to the pandemic, gave rise to feelings of anguish, apathy, lack of future, the end of life as a couple. In the most severe cases, emotionally more vulnerable subjects experienced feelings of escape, suicidal thoughts, or self-harming behaviors.

Many partners reported having even thought it would have been better to be treated for a cancerous disease than for infertility: especially in partners who had dreamed of a family with children since childhood. Alongside this, couples also showed difficulty in making sense of things. Women commonly reported a deterioration of the couple's sexual life because, over time, the purpose of the relationship had become exclusively the achievement of conception and the pandemic had crushed this dream. Partners felt tired and experienced sexuality as a "chore" to avoid, even to the point of thinking about interrupting any kind of sexual and procreative experience. From here arguments, crises, dissatisfaction with the quality of the relationship: annoyance toward the other's body, reluctance in cohabitation, lack of dialogue and confrontation.

The clinical experience, however, has shown in other couples a renewed ability for cohesion and mutual support. A more intense way of experiencing friends and families, a renewed desire for affection and belonging. Certainly, the anguish of death that the pandemic has brought to every human being has led these couples not to give up strong bonds and to be united beyond the threat of COVID-19.

The only regret in both types of couples was the lack of emotional reception and empathic participation on the part of healthcare workers. Even though it was possible to reach them via telemedicine, the approach seemed exclusively clinical. Some noted that doctors too were in mortal danger and often shared the fears, anxieties, fears of that period, with their patients. "It's a shame" reported one post-pandemic couple "that few doctors consulted with mental health professionals. They would have found a part of their own humanity in need of support and help, support and help which they could then have transmitted to us patients."

References

1. Aitken RJ (2022) COVID-19 and male infertility: an update. Andrology 10(1):8–10. https://doi.org/10.1111/andr.13098
2. He Y, Wang J, Ren J, Zhao Y, Chen J, Chen X (2021) Effect of COVID-19 on male reproductive system—a systematic review. Front Endocrinol (Lausanne) 12:677701. https://doi.org/10.3389/fendo.2021.677701
3. Marin L, Ambrosini G, Nuzzi L, Bordin L, Andrisani A (2022) A suggestion to overcome potential risks for infertility due to COVID-19: a response to Aitken. Andrology 10(1):11–12. https://doi.org/10.1111/andr.13100
4. Moreno-Perez O, Merino E, Alfayate R, Torregrosa ME, Andres M, Leon-Ramirez JM, Boix V, Gil J, Pico A, Group CAR;. COVID19-ALC Research Group (2022) Male pituitary-gonadal axis dysfunction in the post-acute COVID-19 syndrome—prevalence and associated factors: a series of Mediterranean cases. Clin Endocrinol 96:353–362
5. Salonia A, Pontillo M, Capogrosso P, Gregori S, Tassara M, Boeri L, Carenzi C, Abbate C, Cignoli D, Ferrara AM et al (2021) Severely low testosterone in males with COVID-19: a case-control study. Andrology 9:1043–1052
6. Yamamoto Y, Otsuka Y, Sunada N, Tokumasu K, Nakano Y, Honda H, Sakurada Y, Hagiya H, Hanayama Y, Otsuka F (2022) Detection of male hypogonadism in patients with post COVID-19 condition. J Clin Med 11:1955
7. Salonia A, Pontillo M, Capogrosso P, Gregori S, Carenzi C, Ferrara AM, Rowe I, Boeri L, Larcher A, Ramirez GA et al (2022) Testosterone in males with COVID-19: a 7-month cohort study. Andrology 10:34–41

8. Scroppo FI, Costantini E, Zucchi A, Illiano E, Trama F, Brancorsini S, Crocetto F, Gismondo MR, Deho F, Mercuriali A et al (2021) COVID-19 disease in the clinical setting: impact on gonadal function, risk of transmission and sperm quality in young males. J Basic Clin Physiol Pharmacol 33:97–102
9. Holtmann N, Edimiris P, Andree M, Doehmen C, Baston-Buest D, Adams O, Kruessel JS, Bielfeld AP (2020) Evaluation of SARS-CoV-2 in human sperm: a cohort study. Fertil Steril 114:233–238
10. Li H, Xiao X, Zhang J, Zafar MI, Wu C, Long Y, Lu W, Pan F, Meng T, Zhao K et al (2020) Altered spermatogenesis in patients with COVID-19. EClinicalMedicine b 28:100604
11. Rambhatla A, Bronkema CJ, Corsi N, Keeley J, Sood A, Affas Z, Dabaja AA, Rogers CG, Liroff SA, Abdollah F (2021) COVID-19 infection in men on testosterone replacement therapy. J Sex Med 18:215–218
12. Li K, Chen G, Hou H, Liao Q, Chen J, Bai H, Lee S, Wang C, Li H, Cheng L et al (2021) Analysis of sexual hormones and menstruation in COVID-19 women of childbearing age. Reproduce Biomed Online 42:260–267
13. Kolanska K, Hours A, Jonquière L, Mathieu d'Argent E, Dabi Y, Dupont C, Touboul C, Antoine JM, Chabbert-Buffet N, Daraï E (2021) Mild COVID-19 infection does not alter ovarian reserve in women treated with ART. Reproduce Biomed Online 43:1117–1121
14. Ding T, Wang T, Zhang J, Cui P, Chen Z, Zhou S, Yuan S, Ma W, Zhang M, Rong Y et al (2021) Analysis of ovarian damage associated with COVID-19 disease in women of reproductive age in Wuhan, China: an observational study. Front Med (Lausanne) 8:635255
15. Bentov Y, Beharier O, Moav-Zafrir A, Kabessa M, Godin M, Greenfield CS, Ketzinel-Gilad M, Ash Broder E, Holzer HEG, Wolf D et al (2021) Ovarian follicular function is not altered by SARS-CoV-2 infection or COVID-19 vaccination with mRNA BNT162b2. Hum Reprod 36:2506–2513
16. Madendag IC, Madendag Y, Ozdemir AT (2022) COVID-19 disease does not cause ovarian lesions in women of reproductive age: an observational study before and after COVID-19. Reproduce Biomed Online 45:153–158
17. Morris RS (2021) Seropositivity to SARS-CoV-2 spike proteins derived from vaccination or infection does not cause sterility. Rep FS 2:253–255
18. Aizer A, Noach-Hirsh M, Dratviman-Storobinsky O, Nahum R, Machtinger R, Yung Y, Haas J, Orvieto R (2022) The effect of immunity to coronavirus disease 2019 on the outcome of frozen-thawed embryo transfer cycles. Fertil Steril 117:974–979
19. ESHRE—(2020) European Society of Human Reproduction and Embryology. Assisted reproduction and COVID-19: a statement from ESHRE for phase 1 of the fertility services guidance during the pandemic. https://www.eshre.eu/Europe/Position-statements/COVID19/#phase1
20. Lambalk CB, van Wely M, Kirkegaard K, Williams AC, de Geyter C (2020) Safety first—assisted human reproduction then. Hum Reprod 35:741–742
21. Veiga A, Gianaroli L, Ory S, Horton M, Feinberg E, Penzias A (2020) Assisted reproduction and COVID-19: a joint statement of ASRM, ESHRE and IFFS. Hum Reprod Open 2020(3):hoaa033. https://doi.org/10.1093/hropen/hoaa033
22. Zaçe D, La Gatta E, Petrella L, Di Pietro ML (2022) The impact of COVID-19 vaccines on fertility-a systematic review and meta-analysis. Vaccine 40(42):6023–6034. https://doi.org/10.1016/j.vaccine.2022.09.019
23. Romer D, Jamieson KH (2020) Conspiracy theories as barriers to controlling the spread of COVID-19 in the US. Soc Sci Med 263:113356. https://doi.org/10.1016/j.socscimed.2020.113356
24. Pinho AC (2020) EMA recommends authorization in the EU for the first COVID-19 vaccine | European Medicines Agency. https://www.ema.europa.eu/en/news/ema-recommends-first-covid-19-vaccine-authorisation-eu
25. The FDA authorizes the Moderna COVID-19 vaccine | The Medical Letter, Inc. 2021. https://secure.medicalletter.org/w1616a

26. Comirnaty and Pfizer-BioNTech COVID-19 Vaccine | FDA. (2021, March 2). https://www.fda.gov/emergency-preparedness-and-response/coronavirus-disease-2019-covid-19/comirnaty-and-pfizer-biontech-covid-19-vaccine
27. Wodarg WSD (1 December 2020) Petition/motion for administrative/regulatory action regarding the confirmation of efficacy endpoints and the use of data in relation to the following clinical studies: phase III-number eudract: 2020–002641-2. corona-ausschuss.de. https://www.wodarg.com/app/download/9033912514/ Wodarg_Yeadon_EMA_Petition_Pfizer_Trial_FINAL_ 01DEC2020_signed_with_Exhibits_geschwa%CC%88rzt.pdf? t=1606870652
28. Aharon D, Lederman M, Ghofranian A, Hernandez-Nieto C, Canon C, Hanley W, Gounko D, Lee JA, Stein D, Buyuk E, Copperman AB (2022) In vitro fertilization and early pregnancy outcomes after coronavirus disease 2019 (COVID-19) vaccination. Obstet Gynecol 139(4):490–497. https://doi.org/10.1097/AOG.0000000000004713. PMID: 35080199
29. Applebaum J, Humphries LA, Kravitz E, Taberski S, Koelper N, Gracia C, Berger DS (2024) Impact of coronavirus disease 2019 vaccination on live birth rates after in vitro fertilization. Fertil Steril 121(3):452–459. https://doi.org/10.1016/j.fertnstert.2023.11.033. Epub 2023 Dec 1. PMID: 38043842
30. Dellazizzo L, Léveillé N, Landry C, Dumais A (2021) Systematic review on the impacts of mental health and COVID-19 treatment on neurocognitive disorders. J Pers Med 11(8):746. https://doi.org/10.3390/JPM11080746
31. Deeks J, Higgins JP, Altman D (2021) Data analysis and conducting meta-analysis. In: JPT H, Thomas J, Chandler J, Cumpston M, Li T, WV PMJ (eds) Cochrane handbook for systematic reviews of interventions version 6.2. Cochrane, pp 1–649
32. Stroup DF, Berlin JA, Morton SC, Olkin I, Williamson GD, Rennie D, Moher D, Becker BJ, Sipe TA, Thacker SB (2000) Meta-analysis of observational studies in epidemiology: a proposal for reporting. JAMA 283:2008. https://doi.org/10.1001/jama.283.15.2008
33. Lablanche O, Salle B, Perie MA, Labrune E, Langlois-Jacques C, Fraison E (2022) Psychological effect of the COVID-19 pandemic among women undergoing infertility treatment, a French cohort—psychological effect PsyCovART of COVID-19: PsyCovART. J Gynecol Obstet Hum Reprod 51:102251. https://doi.org/10.1016/j.jogoh.2021.102251
34. Cirillo M, Rizzello F, Badolato L, De Angelis D, Evangelisti P, Coccia ME, Fatini C (2021) The effects of the COVID-19 lockdown on lifestyle and emotional state in women undergoing assisted reproduction technology: results of an Italian survey. J Gynecol Obstet Hum Reprod 50:102079. https://doi.org/10.1016/j.jogoh.102079
35. Galhardo A, Carolino N, Monteiro B, Cunha M (2022) The emotional impact of the Covid-19 pandemic in women facing infertility. Med Psychological Health 27(2):389–395
36. Mitrović M, Kostić JO, Ristić M (2023) Intolerance to uncertainty and distress in women with delayed IVF treatment due to the COVID-19 pandemic: the mediating role of situation assessment and coping strategies. J Health Psychologist 201:135910532110499
37. Biviá-Roig G, Boldó-Roda A, Blasco-Sanz R, Serrano-Raya L, DelaFuente-Díez E, Múzquiz-Barberá P, Lisón JF (2021) Impact of the COVID-19 pandemic on the lifestyles and quality of life of women with fertility problems: a cross-sectional study. Front Public Health 9:686115. https://doi.org/10.3389/fpubh.2021.686115
38. Dong M, Wu S, Tao Y, Zhou F, Tan J (2021) The impact of postponed fertility treatment on the sexual health of infertile patients owing to the COVID-19 pandemic. Front Med (Lausanne) 8:730994. https://doi.org/10.3389/fmed.2021.730994
39. Jaiswal P, Mahey R, Singh S, Vanamail P, Gupta M, Cheluvaraju R, Sharma JB, Bhatla N (2022) Psychological impact of the suspension/delay of fertility treatments on infertile women waiting during the COVID pandemic. Obstet Gynecol Sci 65:197–206. https://doi.org/10.5468/ogs.21254
40. Rasekh Jahromi A, Daroneh E, Jamali S, Ranjbar A, Rahmanian V (2022) Impact of the COVID-19 pandemic on depression and despair in infertile women. J Psychosom Obstet Gynecol 43:495–501. https://doi.org/10.1080/0167482X.2082279

41. Ben-Kimhy R, Youngster M, Medina-Artom TR, Avraham S, Gat I, Marom Haham L, Hourvitz A, Kedem A (2020) Fertility patients under COVID-19: attitudes, perceptions, and psychological reactions. Hum Reprod (Oxford England) 35:2774–2783. https://doi.org/10.1093/humrep/deaa248
42. Şahin B, Şahin B, Karlı P, Sel G, Hatırnaz Ş, Kara OF, Tinelli A (2021) Level of depression and despair among women with infertility during the COVID-19 epidemic: a cross-sectional survey. Clin Exp Obstet Gynecol 48:594. https://doi.org/10.31083/j.ceog.2021.03.2435
43. Lawson AK, McQueen DB, Swanson AC, Confino R, Feinberg EC, Pavone ME (2021) Psychological distress and deferred fertility care during the COVID-19 pandemic. J Assist Reprod Genet 38:333–341. https://doi.org/10.1007/s10815-020-02023-x
44. Marom Haham L, Youngster M, Kuperman Shani A, Yee S, Ben-Kimhy R, Medina-Artom TR, Hourvitz A, Kedem A, Librach C (2021) Suspension of fertility treatment during the COVID-19 pandemic: opinions, emotional reactions and psychological distress among women undergoing fertility treatments. Reprod Biomed Online 42:849–858. https://doi.org/10.1016/j.rbmo.01.007
45. Dillard AJ, Weber AE, Chassee A, Thakur M (2022) Perceptions of the COVID-19 pandemic among women with infertility: correlations with dispositional optimism. Int J Environ Res Public Health 19:2577. https://doi.org/10.3390/ijerph19052577
46. Biviá-Roig G, Boldó-Roda A, Blasco-Sanz R, Serrano-Raya L, DelaFuente-Díez E, Múzquiz-Barberá P, Lisón JF (2021) Impact of the COVID-19 pandemic on lifestyle and quality of life of women with fertility problems: a cross-sectional study. Front Public Health 9:1–10. https://doi.org/10.3389/fpubh.2021.686115
47. Cao LB, Hao Q, Liu Y, Sun Q, Wu B, Chen L, Yan L (2021) Level of anxiety during the second localized COVID-19 pandemic among infertile women in quarantine: a cross-sectional survey in China. Front Psych 12:1–9. https://doi.org/10.3389/fpsyt.2021.647483
48. Vaughan DA, Shah JS, Penzias AS, Domar AD, Toth TL (2020) Infertility remains one of the main stress factors despite the COVID-19 pandemic. Play Biomed Online 41:425–427. https://doi.org/10.1016/j.rbmo.2020.05.015
49. Grens H, de Bruin JP, Huppelschoten A, Kremer JAM (2022) Fertility workup with video consultation during the COVID-19 pandemic: quantitative and qualitative pilot study. JMIR Formative Res 6:e32000. https://doi.org/10.2196/32000
50. Alhajri N, Simsekler MCE, Alfalasi B, Alhashmi M, AlGhatrif M, Balalaa N, Al Ali M, Almaashari R, Al Memari S, Al Hosani F, Al Zaabi Y, Almazroui S, Alhashemi H, Baltatu OC (2021) Physicians' attitudes toward telemedicine consultations during the COVID-19 pandemic: cross-sectional study. JMIR Med Inform 9(6):e29251. https://doi.org/10.2196/29251
51. Dube L, Nkosi-Mafutha N, Balsom AA, Gordon JL (2021) Infertility-related distress and clinical targets for psychotherapy: a qualitative study. BMJ Open 11(11):e050373. https://doi.org/10.1136/bmjopen-2021-050373

Chapter 7
Endometriosis, Infertility, and Sexuality

Scientific literature shows that one in nine women suffers from endometriosis [1]: a chronic inflammatory condition characterized by chronic pelvic pain, fatigue, dysmenorrhea (painful menstruation), dyspareunia (pain associated with sexual intercourse), nausea, and intestinal and bladder problems [2]. Patients living with endometriosis (ILWE) experience significant diagnostic delays of about 6–8 years after the onset of symptoms [3]. Moreover, severe symptoms often recur even following invasive surgical procedures [3].

A recent study by Gete et al. [4] examined 3728 women with endometriosis, born between 1973 and 1978, using data from the Australian Longitudinal Study on Women's Health. To examine the association between endometriosis and health-related quality of life (HRQoL) scales were used, comparing women who had a lower HRQoL (score below the 25th percentile) with those who had a higher HRQoL (score above the 25th percentile). Women's HRQoL was assessed using the Short Form Survey of 36 items every 3 years from 1996 to 2018.

Results: Endometriosis was associated with significantly worse HRQoL scores over time. In comparison with women without endometriosis, patients with endometriosis showed worse scores in physical functioning 1.33 (1.19, 1.50), role physical 1.57 (1.41, 1.74), bodily pain 1.65 (1.48, 1.82), general health 1.61 (1.42, 1.81), vitality 1.38 (1.23, 1.55), social functioning 1.38 (1.25, 1.53), role emotional 1.19 (1.06, 1.33), mental health 1.32 (1.18, 1.48). Women with endometriosis also had significantly lower scores on physical health 1.68 (1.51, 1.88) and mental health components 1.28 (1.14, 1.44).

This is compounded by infertility.

Currently, infertility associated with endometriosis is seen as a multifactorial problem (including factors related to altered immunity and genetics), which affects not only the fallopian tubes and the embryo transport but also the normal endometrium [5]. At present, the treatment of infertility caused by endometriosis focuses on the removal or reduction of ectopic endometrial implants and restoring normal pelvic anatomy through medical, surgical, or assisted reproduction technology means

E. V. Longhi, *Framing Sexual Dysfunctions and Diseases during Fertility Treatment*, https://doi.org/10.1007/978-3-031-76726-5_7

[6]. The medical approach targets ovarian function, blocking it with various drugs such as gonadotropin-releasing hormone agonists and oral contraceptives. Assisted reproduction technologies (ART), like in vitro fertilization (IVF), come into play when neither the medical nor surgical attempts achieve the desired result. It has been shown that in vitro fertilization represents one of the key therapeutic options for patients suffering from infertility associated with endometriosis, especially when it involves a compromised tubal function, compromised peritoneal anatomy, or the failure of other treatment methods [7].

The causes of infertility in women with endometriosis can vary from anatomical distortions due to adhesions and fibrosis to endocrine abnormalities and immunological disorders. In some cases, the various pathophysiological disorders seem to interact through mechanisms not yet fully understood. Medical or hormonal treatment alone has little or no effect and should only be used in combination with assisted reproduction technology (ART). Among the various methods of ART, intrauterine insemination, for its simplicity, can be recommended for women with minimal or mild peritoneal endometriosis, even though insemination may produce a lower success rate compared to women without endometriosis. In vitro fertilization (IVF) is an effective treatment option in the less advanced stages of the disease and the success rates are similar to the results in other causes of infertility. However, women with more advanced stages of endometriosis have lower success rates with in vitro fertilization.

The study by Federica Facchin et al. [8], conducted at the Infertility Unit of the Fondazione Ca′ Granda, Ospedale Maggiore Policlinico in Milan between 2017 and 2018, included 269 patients with infertility aged between 24 and 45 years (37.8 ± 4.0 years). The outcomes of sexual function were sexual dysfunction (assessed with the Female Sexual Function Index), sexual distress (assessed with the Female Sexual Distress Scale-Revised), dyspareunia, and the number of intercourses in the month prior to ovarian stimulation. The distress related to infertility was measured with the Fertility Problem Inventory (FPI). Demographic variables (age and level of education of women and their partners) and factors related to infertility were also examined, such as the type and concurrent causes of infertility, the number of previous in vitro fertilization cycles, and duration of infertility.

Results: Women with greater distress related to infertility were more likely to report sexual dysfunction (odds ratio = 1.02 per score point; 95% CI, 1.01–1.03; $P = 0.001$). Three FPI domains (social, relational, and sexual concerns) were correlated with almost all outcomes of sexual function ($P < 0.05$).

The limitation of this study was that sexually active women were not included as there was a lack of information on the sexual function of partners and the resulting distress due to infertility.

However, we still have a series of specific studies on these topics [9]. A systematic literature search was performed to identify studies that evaluated sexual function in patients with endometriosis and a narrative analysis of the results is presented. The review discusses important quantitative and qualitative studies that analyze the effects of endometriosis and its hormonal and surgical treatments on measures of sexual function and the quality of the sexual relationship, as well as the resulting infertility.

To reach an attempt at ART, patients with endometriosis have undergone years of sexual experiences associated with pain and fear of pain. The fear reaction in turn negatively influences desire, arousal, orgasm, lubrication, loss of genital congestion, and an increase in pelvic floor tone in a circular model [10]. Furthermore, anxiety, bitterness, or frustration during or following sexual intercourse and feelings of guilt and distress negatively affect the hypothesis of a positive parental outcome because it is conditioned by catastrophic feelings of failure and despair. Finally, central sensitization leads to hyperalgesia and allodynia and secondary hyperalgesia and worsening of pain perception [11].

In conclusion, based on the available albeit limited evidence (the first studies date back to 1995), endometriosis seems to have an impact on all areas of sexual function, desire/arousal, orgasm, satisfaction, and pain, leading to sexual dysfunction and discomfort in 70–75% of patients, at least in advanced stages. Repetitive painful experiences with a negative outcome, probably shift the sexual response from motivation/arousal to hypervigilance and from desire to fear and avoidance, leading to sexual discomfort in symptomatic endometriosis patients. Consequently, the partners show disappointment, anger, restlessness, and a submission toward more affectionate than erotic practices, which are often rejected by the partner. During ART, sexuality is nullified and the couple becomes relationally competitive and symbiotic. In case of positive outcome of ART, sexuality is nullified and the partner mostly turns to self-eroticism, passive pornographic viewing, and occasional commercial sex to compensate for the void in the couple's sexuality.

7.1 Her Pain, His Frustration

Thus, dyspareunia, female sexual dysfunction, and associated infertility compromise the relationship with the partner and his sexual functioning, especially in young couples. Erectile dysfunction or premature ejaculation are the most frequent dysfunctions. The fear of causing the partner pain with penetration often leads partners to protect her, attributing a difficulty in the sexual response. In this case, the frustration between the partners becomes a common condition.

At this point, sexuality is not even discussed [12]. In the study WERF Endocost, among women in relationships, 67% reported significant problems with their partner caused by endometriosis (34% of women) and 19% of women considered endometriosis to be the cause of divorce (10% of women). It seems that 15% of women with endometriosis reported having had serious relationship problems for a period of 15 years and 7.7% have suffered from a relationship interrupted due to the symptoms of endometriosis [13].

But there is more.

According to the cognitive behavioral model [14], these body changes induced by the disease activate negative automatic thoughts, related to the physical aspect, maladaptive behaviors, and emotional discomfort. In qualitative research, patients expressed frustration, feelings of despair, and loss of confidence regarding the limits and changes that endometriosis imposes on their bodies [15]. The swelling and weight gain, particularly during "flare-ups" of symptoms, make patients unable to wear their favorite clothes, both to avoid physical discomfort and to hide body features considered embarrassing and socially undesirable [16].

In the face of such behaviors, many partners, already frustrated by an almost absent sexuality and an unlikely desire for parenthood, tend to emotionally distance themselves, to devote themselves entirely to work, sports, and personal interests, until they feel a sense of distressing relational imprisonment and a desire to escape. The loneliness of both partners is not always evaluated as a couple. It is always the patient who is evaluated more deeply. These are the most used questionnaires:

The De Jong-Giervel Loneliness Scale (DJGLS) more often evaluates women with social loneliness [17] (e.g., "there are enough people I feel close to") and emotional loneliness (e.g., "I often feel rejected," "I miss having a really dear friend"). Total scores range from 0 to 5 (social) and from 0 to 6 (emotional), with higher scores indicating greater feelings of loneliness. The subscale of the social support of the Endometriosis Health Profile 30 (EHP-30) [18] evaluated the perceived social support (e.g., "Did you feel like others thought you were complaining?", "Did you not feel able to tell people how you feel?"). Developed using interviews with ILWE, the EHP-30 is a frequently used measure of the quality of life specific to endometriosis: it consists of four items and is converted into a total score out of 100, representing the lowest level of perceived social support [19]. The Body Image Scale (BIS) [20] evaluates the cognitive, behavioral, and affective aspects of body image (e.g., "Are you satisfied with your appearance when you are dressed?", "Did you feel uncomfortable about your appearance?"). Originally developed in an oncological context, it has since been used in endometriosis [21]. An item related to feelings of femininity was removed to ensure gender inclusion. Scores higher than 30 indicate a worse body image and scores equal to or greater than 10 denote a probably clinically significant BIS [22]. Subsequently, the quality of sleep was investigated: Pittsburgh Sleep Quality Index (PSQI) [23]. This questionnaire contains 19 items in seven areas (sleep quality, sleep latency, sleep duration, habitual sleep efficiency, sleep disturbances, use of sleeping medication, and daytime dysfunction) on a scale from 0 to 3; therefore, the total PSQI score ranges from 0 to 21. A total score above 5 identifies poor QS and scores below 5 show absence of sleep disorders.

As far as scientific research is concerned, more consideration needs to be given to intersex people and the circumstances of a state of infertility that can be traced during childhood, girlhood, or adolescence, before or outside attempts at conception and without undergoing fertility treatments. The perspective of scientific research is moving toward verifying the state of infertility in combination with an atypical sexual state in the early stages of life. However, infertility is not considered pathological or constantly prohibitive for the entire life of all affected people. The perceptions of intersex women of a potentially childless future are varied, complex, ambivalent, and, in some cases, transitory throughout the course of life.

But there is more.

Diagnosis plays an important role in health and medicine. As Sim and Madden [24] argue, "diagnosis is not simply a tool" used by doctors to prescribe treatments and predict prognoses; it is rather a social and political mechanism that has significant repercussions on identity and on the meaning and understanding of disease. For example, a diagnosis gives people permission to assume the role of a patient. It legitimizes their feelings and their actions. In this way, diagnoses can remove individual blame by instead blaming the etiology of the disease [25]. Madden and Sim [26] have also found that diagnoses allow individuals to regain control over their own disease by removing uncertainty and allowing adaptation.

7.2 Conclusions [27]

In conclusion, intrauterine insemination (IUI) and in vitro fertilization (IVF) improve pregnancy rates, but women with endometriosis have lower pregnancy rates compared to patients with other causes of infertility. The decision whether to operate or pursue assisted reproduction will depend on a number of factors such as the patient's symptoms, the presence of complex masses on ultrasound, ovarian reserve and ovarian access for in vitro fertilization, the risk of surgery, and the costs.

Regarding the influence of endometriosis on women's physical and mental health, it is not unlikely that the greatest impact of endometriosis on sexual dysfunction is exerted by anxiety, depression, sleep quality, pelvic pain, and dyspareunia. Despite this, the potentially harmful impacts of pelvic pain and dyspareunia, the stage of endometriosis, educational status, physical activity, and BMI can influence the SF.

The evaluation of a medically assisted path for infertility represents a further ordeal for the patient and the partner. This indicates that in the care of women with endometriosis, not only should laparoscopy and medical treatment be performed, but also psychotherapeutic and psychosexual help be offered. For Her, for Him, for the couple. Partners appear completely disoriented already at the first gynecological evaluation of the partner. Impotence, the sense of inadequacy most often felt, induces in partners ambivalent feelings: from excessive care, to abandonment, to resentment. Taking care of the partner from the beginning of any clinical path, including infertility, would make the feelings of fatigue, suffering, and nullity of each individual more evident. Reserving for them an individualized and exculpatory accompaniment, a useful tool to ensure that no one deprives themselves of a life project.

References

1. Rowlands I, Abbott J, Montgomery G, Hockey R, Rogers P, Mishra G (2021) Prevalence and incidence of endometriosis in Australian women: a data linkage cohort study. BJOG Int J Gynaecol Obstet 128:657–665
2. Becker K, Heinemann K, Imthurn B, Marions L, Moehner S, Gerlinger C, Serrani M, Faustmann T (2021) Real world data on symptomology and diagnostic approaches of 27,840 women living with endometriosis. Sci Rep 11(1):20404. https://doi.org/10.1038/s41598-021-99681-3
3. Nnoaham KE, Hummelshoj L, Webster P, d'Hooghe T, de Cicco NF, de Cicco NC, Jenkinson C, Kennedy SH, Zondervan KT, World Endometriosis Research Foundation Global Study of Women's Health consortium (2011) Impact of endometriosis on quality of life and work productivity: a multicenter study across ten countries. Fertil Steril 96(2):366–373.e8. https://doi.org/10.1016/j.fertnstert.2011.05.090
4. Gete DG, Doust J, Mortlock S, Montgomery G, Mishra GD (2023) Impact of endometriosis on women's health-related quality of life: a national prospective cohort study. Maturitas 174:1–7. https://doi.org/10.1016/j.maturitas.2023.04.272. Epub 2023 May 6. PMID: 37182389
5. Macer ML, Taylor HS (2012) Endometriosis and infertility: a review of the pathogenesis and treatment of endometriosis-associated infertility. Obstet Gynecol Clin N Am 39(4):535–549. https://doi.org/10.1016/j.ogc.2012.10.002
6. Dunselman GA, Vermeulen N, Becker C, Calhaz-Jorge C, D'Hooghe T, De Bie B, Heikinheimo O, Horne AW, Kiesel L, Nap A, Prentice A, Saridogan E, Soriano D, Nelen W, European Society of Human Reproduction and Embryology (2014) ESHRE guideline: management of women with endometriosis. Hum Reprod 29(3):400–412. https://doi.org/10.1093/humrep/det457
7. Opoien HK, Fedorcsak P, Omland AK, Abyholm T, Bjercke S, Ertzeid G, Oldereid N, Mellembakken JR, Tanbo T (2012) In vitro fertilization is an effective treatment in infertility associated with endometriosis. Fertil Steril 97:912–918. https://doi.org/10.1016/j.fertnstert.2012.01.112
8. Facchin F, Somigliana E, Busnelli A, Catavorello A, Barbara G, Vercellini P (2019) Infertility-related distress and female sexual function during assisted reproduction. Hum Reprod 34(6):1065–1073. https://doi.org/10.1093/humrep/dez046
9. Pluchino N, Wenger JM, Petignat P, Tal R, Bolmont M, Taylor HS, Bianchi-Demicheli F (2016) Sexual function in endometriosis patients and their partners: effect of the disease and consequences of treatment. Hum Reprod Update 22(6):762–774. https://doi.org/10.1093/humupd/dmw031
10. Payne KA, Binik YM, Amsel R, Khalifé S (2005) When sex hurts, anxiety and fear orient attention towards pain. Eur J Pain 9(4):427–436. https://doi.org/10.1016/j.ejpain.2004.10.003
11. Thomtén J, Lundahl R, Stigenberg K, Linton S (2014) Fear avoidance and pain catastrophizing among women with sexual pain. Womens Health (Lond) 10(6):571–581. https://doi.org/10.2217/whe.14.51
12. Vitale SG, La Rosa VL, Rapisarda AMC, Laganà AS (2017) Endometriosis and infertility: the impact on quality of life and mental health. J Endometriosis Pelvic Pain Disord 9(2):112–115
13. Sorensen J, Bautista KE, Lamvu G, Feranec J (2018) Evaluation and treatment of female sexual pain: a clinical review. Cureo 10(3):e2379
14. Melis I, Litta P, Nappi L, Agus M, Melis GB, Angioni S (2015) Sexual function in women with deep endometriosis: correlation with quality of life, pain intensity, depression, anxiety and body image. Int J Sexual Health 27:175–185
15. Roomaney R, Kagee A (2018) Salient aspects of quality of life among women diagnosed with endometriosis: a qualitative study. J Health Psychologist 23:905–916
16. Jones G, Jenkinson C, Kennedy S (2004) The impact of endometriosis on quality of life: a qualitative analysis. J Psychosom Obstet Gynaecol 25:123–133
17. De Jong-Gierveld J, Kamphuls F (1985) The development of a Rasch-type loneliness scale. Appl Psychol Measure 9:289–299

18. Jones G, Kennedy S, Barnard A, Wong J, Jenkinson C (2001) Development of an endometriosis quality of life instrument: the Endometriosis Health Profile-30. Obstet Gynecol 98:258–264
19. Bourdel N, Chauvet P, Billone V, Douridas G, Fauconnier A, Gerbaud L, Canis M (2019) Systematic review of quality of life measures in patients with endometriosis. PLoS One 14(1):e0208464. https://doi.org/10.1371/journal.pone.0208464
20. Hopwood P, Fletcher I, Lee A, Al GS (2001) A body image scale for use with cancer patients. Eur J Cancer 37:189–197
21. Pehlivan MJ, Sherman KA, Wuthrich V, Horn M, Basson M, Duckworth T (2022) Body image and depression in endometriosis: examination of self-esteem and rumination as mediators. Body Image 43:463–473
22. Chopra D, De La Garza R, Lacourt TE (2021) Clinical relevance of a cut-off point of 10 on the body image scale as an indicator of psychological distress in patients with cancer: results from a psychiatric oncology clinic. Support Care Cancer 29:231–237
23. Moghaddam JF, Nakhaee N, Sheibani V, Garrusi B, Amirkafi A (2012) Reliability and validity of the Persian version of the Pittsburgh Sleep Quality Index (PSQI-P). Sleep Breath 16(1):79–82. https://doi.org/10.1007/s11325-010-0478-5
24. Sim J, Madden S (2008) Illness experience in the fibromyalgia syndrome: a metasynthesis of qualitative studies. Soc Sci Med 67(1):57–67
25. Arksey H, Sloper P (1999) Contested diagnoses: the cases of RSI and childhood cancer. Soc Sci Med 49(4):483–497
26. Madden S, Sim J (2006) Creating meaning in fibromyalgia syndrome. Soc Sci Med 63(11):2962–2973
27. Youseflu S, Jahanian Sadatmahalleh S, Bahri Khomami M, Nasiri M (2020) Influential factors on sexual function in infertile women with endometriosis: a path analysis. BMC Womens Health 20(1):92. https://doi.org/10.1186/s12905-020-00941-7

Chapter 8
Bleeding and Miscarriage

A threat to the desire for parenthood.

The desire for parenthood is often conditioned by humiliating and painful events experienced by the infertile couple: sudden bleeding, a miscarriage.

Disappointment, anger, depression, a sense of injustice, persecution, suffering, guilt toward the partner, withdrawal from the world: these are the most recurring feelings after traumatic events such as a failed pregnancy. Even the emotional intimacy between partners seems too much and every hug can be experienced as a threat, an improper act, and an inexplicable abuse.

If miscarriages become more than an isolated event, then we speak of recurrent miscarriages (RM). They are defined by at least three episodes of consecutive miscarriages (RM) of less than 14 weeks of amenorrhea (SA), with the same partner, in a patient under 40 years old. These patients present in 80% of cases an identifiable cause that justifies an etiological approach: anatomical, chromosomal, endocrinological, thrombophilic, immunological, and idiopathic causes [1].

The Study Group of the Abortive Disease (GEMA), created in 2004, uses the following definition for recurrent miscarriages (RM), while the frequency of an "isolated" miscarriage is estimated at 15% and the probability of resulting in three consecutive miscarriages would therefore be 0.3%.

RM requires an etiological assessment to determine the causes that benefit from a treatment likely to reduce the risk of recurrence.

Ongoing research on other possible etiologies of RM has highlighted immune mechanisms, identifiable in particular through natural killer (NK) lymphocytes and TH17. In fact, NK lymphocytes are reported to be involved in the mechanisms of immune tolerance of semi-allogeneic grafts such as pregnancy.

However, although recurrent miscarriage may be associated with endocrine, anatomical, psychological, infectious, thrombotic, genetic, or immunological causes, over 50% of cases remain unexplained, even after a thorough diagnosis. The frequency with which sperm defects contribute to recurrent miscarriage has not been

E. V. Longhi, *Framing Sexual Dysfunctions and Diseases during Fertility Treatment*, https://doi.org/10.1007/978-3-031-76726-5_8

established [2], and the relationship between standard sperm parameters and recurrent miscarriages is a controversial topic [3].

The study by Sbracia et al. [3] investigated the role of the "male factor" in the pathogenesis of recurrent spontaneous abortion (RSA) (particularly sperm morphology anomalies) and recruited 120 couples previously selected with unexplained RSA.

Patients were divided into three subgroups, depending on their reproductive outcome during the 3-year follow-up study:

1. 48 RSA couples who successfully achieved a pregnancy;
2. 39 RSA couples who suffered further miscarriages;
3. 33 RSA couples who experienced infertility during the follow-up period.

A sperm analysis was performed twice at the time of inclusion in the study and again twice during the 3-year follow-up period. No significant differences were observed in sperm parameters between RSA males and fertile controls.

However, significant differences were observed between the group of RSA couples who experienced infertility during follow-up and the other two groups (RSA couples who successfully achieved pregnancy and RSA couples who had spontaneous abortions and no live births during follow-up) for sperm concentration, sperm motility, and sperm morphological abnormalities.

Results: Morphological abnormalities of sperm do not seem to be involved in determining RSA; they instead constitute an etiological factor in determining patient infertility, along with other seminal parameters, in the subsequent reproductive life of the RSA couple.

The partners of patients with recurrent abortions show a significant increase in sperm chromosome aneuploidy, abnormal chromatin condensation, DNA fragmentation, increased apoptosis, and abnormal sperm morphology compared to fertile men.

8.1 His Bad Habits

But there is more.

The relationship between current use of cigarettes, marijuana, and alcohol with the parameters of seminal fluid analysis, sperm penetration test, and sperm autoimmunity was studied in 164 men from infertile couples by Close et al. [4].

Current cigarette smokers, marijuana users, and heavy alcohol consumers showed a higher number of leukocytes in the seminal fluid compared to nonconsumers ($p < 0.02$, < 0.007, and < 0.01, respectively).

In addition, cigarette smokers showed lower scores in the sperm penetration test compared to nonsmokers (median 2.5 vs. 8.0, $p = 0.05$).

Users of cigarettes, marijuana, or alcohol showed no decrease in sperm count, motility, or percentage of oval sperm, and no difference in the prevalence of antisperm antibodies compared to nonusers.

After controlling for past sexually transmitted diseases and multiple exposures to substances in a multivariate model, the use of cigarettes, marijuana, or alcohol continued to be associated with a trend toward an increase in fluid leukocytes in the sperm. Cigarette smoking continued to show a significant decrease in the sperm penetration test score ($p = 0.03$).

Furthermore, the study by Rodriguez-Rigau et al. [5] evaluated the quality of sperm in 437 male partners of infertile couples seen consecutively, excluding 181 men who had factors that could influence sperm quality.

Ninety-seven men affected by varicocele were considered separately.

Of the remaining 159 men, 101 were nonsmokers and 58 were smokers, with an average age of about 31 years.

The average percentage of normal sperm was 44.7% for the group of 101 nonsmokers and 44.8% for the group of smokers. The average sperm motility, the average sperm count, and the frequency distribution of sperm were not very different between the two groups.

The number of cigarettes smoked per day was not a significant factor. The group of 97 men with varicocele analyzed separately showed no differences between smokers and nonsmokers, even though compared to the group of 159 men without varicocele, a significantly higher percentage of men with varicocele had a sperm count of 20 million/mL. It is difficult to explain the differences between these results and those that claim that smoking affects sperm quality.

8.2 Sleep and Pregnancy Clinical Outcome

Sleep disorders are presumed to be common in patients undergoing fertility treatments and a review on the subject has recommended further studies on prevalences and possible associations [6].

According to research conducted worldwide, women who receive assisted reproduction technologies may suffer from somatic and psychological symptoms and have sleep disorders.

Apparently, the guilt of infertility and lack of restful sleep forces Asian women to hide this scenario and delay the moment when they accept medical assistance and mental support.

A longitudinal study by Lin et al. [7] studied 100 infertile female patients who received oocyte retrieval therapies and in vitro fertilization–embryo transfer in a hospital in northern Taiwan. The data were collected through a structured questionnaire, including somatic symptoms, Pittsburgh Sleep Quality Index, and a five-item Brief Symptom Rating Scale. The data were analyzed using the McNemar test, Wilcoxon Sign Rank, and fully entered into multiple regression with SPSS version 20.0 software.

Results: The average age of 100 participants was 34·54 years. They manifested abdominal distension, breast engorgement, nausea, fainting, diarrhea, sleep disorders, and psychological discomfort when they received in vitro fertilization–embryo transfer; these results were apparently higher than for those who had received oocyte retrieval.

Furthermore, sleep disorders were the most significant factor involved in psychological discomfort during oocyte retrieval and in vitro fertilization–embryo transfer therapies. The most severe indicator of women's psychological discomfort during oocyte retrieval and in vitro fertilization–embryo transfer treatment was anxiety.

In summary, sleep disorders represented the most significant factor involved in the psychological discomfort of women who showed conception problems. Relevance for clinical practice, nurses dealing with assisted reproduction technologies can assess women's psychological discomfort by taking care of their sleep disorders without directly exploring their mood. Furthermore, clinicians in general should understand that the psychological discomfort of infertile patients is mainly associated with sleep disorders.

The study by Lateef et al. [8] has shown that sleep patterns condition the synthesis, secretion, and metabolism of hormones necessary for reproduction. Sleep deprivation among men and women is increasingly reported as one of the causes of infertility and miscarriages.

In animal models, sleep disorders compromise the secretion of sex hormones, leading to a decrease in testosterone levels, reduced sperm motility, and apoptosis of Leydig cells in male rats. Sleep deprivation generates intrinsically stressful stimuli, due to circadian desynchrony and therefore increases the activation of the hypothalamus–pituitary–adrenal (HPA) axis, which, consequently, increases the production of corticosterone. The high level of corticosteroids causes a reduction in testosterone production.

Sleep deprivation has a proportional effect on women, reducing chances of fertility. Insomnia among shift workers suppresses the production of melatonin as well as excessive activation of the HPA axis resulting in early pregnancy termination, failed embryo implantation, anovulation, and amenorrhea.

It has been found that sleep deprivation in women is also associated with altered secretion of gonadotropins and sex steroids, both of which lead to female infertility. In men with poor sleep quality, low concentrations of testosterone are evident.

8.3 Miscarriage: What Is It?

In the event of a miscarriage, two conditions can occur: the miscarriage can be complete, with total expulsion by the body of the product of conception and the placenta and relative emptying of the uterus or incomplete, with the need to intervene with a specific treatment. In cases where part of the placenta or fetal tissues remain in the uterus, one can proceed either through drug treatment with the aim of inducing labor and the consequent expulsion of the contents of the uterus or through a surgical procedure (aspiration curettage). The scientific literature shows how, especially in the case of spontaneous abortion, there are enormous difficulties in terms of post-traumatic stress and risk of depression and anxiety that can persist even in the years following the event.

It has been shown that postabortion is also associated with difficulty in managing the needs of a child of a subsequent and possible pregnancy. Moreover, the pain of the loss seems irreversible and permanently present in the couple's emotions.

Men, on the other hand, can be victims of the sense of loss of a desired child or of a suffered pregnancy because it is mostly conditioned by Her desire. The discordant choices between the two partners can be a source of tension, suffering, and separation for both the man and the woman, leading to profound consequences and which are often too little considered. Separations, divorces, or the search for external relationships often seem like a "magical solution" for both partners, to erase failure and have a second life project. With or without children. However, the basic relationship between the two becomes increasingly ambivalent and manipulative.

8.4 Conclusions

Nevertheless, the failure of in vitro fertilization treatment after a certain number of cycles can be devastating for couples, especially when one or more spontaneous abortions are present.

Although in vitro fertilization strategies try to reduce the psychological burden of treatment, failure can cause feelings of regret for not having adopted a more aggressive approach, including the transfer of two embryos.

The lack of parenthood induces a deep rejection of sexuality in both partners and, in some cases, even body dysmorphia.

A real "war against an inadequate body," unfit, incapable of generating, and being in itself an element of seduction.

The study by Allen J. Wilcox, MD, Ph.D. focused on stress, after two or more implant cycles and a series of spontaneous abortions.

The patients, randomized in two centers, had undergone mild ovarian stimulation and single embryo transfer ($n = 197$) or long protocol ovarian stimulation with standard GnRH agonists with double embryo transfer ($n = 194$).

The patients completed the hospital anxiety and depression scale before starting treatment and 1 week after the outcome of the final treatment cycle was known.

Data from women undergoing two or more cycles of in vitro fertilization ($n = 253$) were analyzed.

Results: Women who experienced therapeutic failure after standard IVF treatment had more symptoms of depression 1 week after the end of treatment than women who had undergone mild IVF.

It can be inferred that the failure of in vitro fertilization treatment after a mild treatment strategy may result in fewer symptoms of short-term depression compared to failure after a standard treatment strategy. This failure of in vitro fertilization treatment after a certain number of cycles can be devastating and irreversible for many couples.

8.5 Celiac Disease, Infertility, and Abortions

For a broader analysis, we must also not forget the effects of celiac disease. It can indeed reduce fertility or complicate pregnancy. The study by Kolho et al. [9] examined women with recurrent abortion of unknown etiology ($n = 63$), unexplained infertility ($n = 47$), and infertility with known cause ($n = 82$) for anti-endomysium antibodies in the serum to find undiagnosed celiac disease. A woman (1–6%) with recurrent abortion, another woman (2.1%) with unexplained infertility, and a woman (2.0%) in the control group ($n = 51$) were considered to have celiac disease. It is hypothesized that a higher frequency of celiac disease in women with infertility or recurrent abortions often remains submerged and undiagnosed.

Celiac disease (CD), also known as "gluten-sensitive enteropathy," is an immune-mediated inflammatory disease of the small intestine; it is triggered by exposure to dietary gluten, derived from wheat, barley, and rye, in genetically predisposed individuals, with an approximate global seroprevalence rate of 1.4% [10].

The female-to-male ratio of Crohn's disease based on serological screening is 1.5:1 and its diagnosis can be quite difficult, as most cases are asymptomatic, while clinical manifestations among symptomatic individuals are quite heterogeneous [11].

A systematic literature search on Medline, Cochrane Library, and Scopus was conducted from the beginning until April 12, 2022, to identify studies that reported the risk of adverse pregnancy outcomes in women with Crohn's disease. The key questions were formulated according to the PICO method: "Do pregnant women diagnosed with celiac disease have a higher risk of adverse pregnancy outcomes compared to pregnant women without celiac disease?" To perform the searches, medical topic words were used: "celiac disease," "CD," "gluten enteropathy,, "pregnancy," "premature," "obstetric," "complication," "preterm birth," "miscarriage spontaneous," "preeclampsia," "gestational hypertension," "stillborn," "cesarean delivery," "postpartum hemorrhage," "gestational diabetes," "placental abruption," "small for gestational age," and "fetal growth restriction" [12].

Results: Based on data from four cohort studies [13] among 5399 pregnancies of women with Crohn's disease and 14,882,102 control pregnancies, there were respectively 134 (2.5%) and 511,846 (3.4%) cases of preeclampsia (or gestosis, a condition that can occur during pregnancy or postpartum and affects both mother and child).

In four cohort studies and two case–control studies [14] comprising 10,011 pregnancies in the CD group and 443,354 cases in the control group, the incidence of stillbirth was 0.58% ($n = 58$) in the study group compared to 0.41% ($n = 1819$) in the control group. The analysis showed a statistically significant correlation between CD and stillbirth (RR 1.57, 95% CI 1.17–2.10).

Nine cohort studies [13] evaluated the risk of PTD among women with Crohn's disease. Overall, the study group consisted of 8012 cases and the control group of 19,437,859 cases, with respectively 582 (7.3%) and 1,197,460 (6.2%) PTD (preterm birth) events. A statistically significant association between CD and PTD was identified.

The meta-analysis of eight cohort studies and one case–control study [13] showed that 1367 (16.9%) out of 8090 women with celiac disease and 4,169,957 (23.2%) women out of 17,953,735 in the control group underwent cesarean delivery. A statistically significant association between CD and cesarean delivery was observed (RR 1.10, 95% CI 1.03–1.16).

In four cohort studies [15], 5216 cases with CD and 15,025,256 controls were included, and postpartum hemorrhage occurred in 183 (3.5%) and 411,727 (2.7%) cases, respectively.

Four cohort studies and one case–control study reported the average body weight of the newborn [16] composed respectively of 1829 and 1,652,997 cases in the study and control groups. Pregnancies of mothers with CD had a statistically significant correlation with a lower average body weight of the newborn.

In summary:

1. The risk of miscarriage, fetal growth restriction, stillbirth, preterm birth, cesarean delivery, and low birth weight was significantly higher in the CD group, compared to the control group without CD.
2. Only pregnant women with undiagnosed Crohn's disease were at high risk of delayed fetal growth, stillbirth, preterm birth, and low birth weight; those diagnosed early did not have a higher risk for the above outcomes, compared to the general pregnant population.
3. Early diagnosis of Crohn's disease minimizes the risk of fetal growth restriction, stillbirth, preterm birth, and low birth weight, possibly through the adoption of a non-diet diet.

References

1. Lepage J, Luton D, Azria E (2015) Aborti spontanei a ripetizione, EMC—AKOS—Trattato di. Medicina 17(3):1–8. https://doi.org/10.1016/S1634-7358(15)72342-9
2. American Society for Reproductive Medicine (ASRM) (2005) Recurrent miscarriages in pregnancy. Patient Fact Sheet. Available at: http://www.asrm.org/Patients/FactSheets/fact.html
3. Sbracia S, Cozza G, Grasso JA, Mastrone M, Scarpellini F (2008) Seminal parameters and sperm morphology in men undergoing unexplained recurrent spontaneous miscarriage, before and during a 3-year follow-up period. Hum Reprod 11(1996):117–120
4. Close CE, Roberts PL, Berger RE (2010) Cigarettes, alcohol and marijuana are related to pyospermia in infertile men. J Urol 144(4):900–903. https://doi.org/10.1016/s0022-5347(17)39618-0
5. Rodriguez-Rigau LJ, Smith KD, Steinberger E (1982) Cigarette smoking and semen quality. Fertil Steril 38(1):115–116. https://doi.org/10.1016/s0015-0282(16)46408-3
6. Kloss JD, Perlis ML, Zamzow JA, Culnan EJ, Grazia CR (2015) Sleep, sleep disorders and fertility in women. Sleep Med Rev 22:78–87
7. Lin YH, Chueh KH, Lin JL (2016) Somatic symptoms, sleep disturbance and psychological distress among women undergoing oocyte pick-up and in vitro fertilisation-embryo transfer. J Clin Nurs 25(11–12):1748–1756. https://doi.org/10.1111/jocn.13194

8. Lateef OM, Akintubosun MO (2020) Sleep and reproductive health. J Circadian Rhythms 18:1. https://doi.org/10.5334/jcr.190
9. Kolho KL, Tiitinen A, Tulppala M, Unkila-Kallio L, Savilahti E (1999) Screening for coeliac disease in women with a history of recurrent miscarriage or infertility. Br J Obstet Gynaecol 106(2):171–173. https://doi.org/10.1111/j.1471-0528.1999.tb08218.x
10. Singh P, Arora A, Strand TA, Leffler DA, Catassi C, Green PH, Kelly CP, Ahuja V, Makharia GK (2018) Global prevalence of celiac disease: systematic review and meta-analysis. Clin Gastroenterol Hepatol 16(6):823–836.e2. https://doi.org/10.1016/j.cgh.2017.06.037
11. Choung RS, Ditah IC, Nadeau AM, Rubio-Tapia A, Marietta EV, Brantner TL, Camilleri MJ, Rajkumar SV, Landgren O, Everhart JE, Murray JA (2015) Trends and racial/ethnic disparities in gluten-sensitive problems in the United States: findings from the National Health and Nutrition Examination Surveys from 1988 to 2012. Am J Gastroenterol 110(3):455–461. https://doi.org/10.1038/ajg.2015.8
12. Arvanitakis K, Siargkas A, Germanidis G, Dagklis T, Tsakiridis I (2023) Adverse pregnancy outcomes in women with celiac disease: a systematic review and meta-analysis. Ann Gastroenterol 36(1):12–24. https://doi.org/10.20524/aog.2022.0764. Epub 2022 Dec 8
13. Elliott B, Czuzoj-Shulman N, Spence AR, Mishkin DS, Abenhaim HA (2021) Effect of celiac disease on maternal and neonatal outcomes of pregnancy. J Matern Fetal Neonatal Med 34:2117–2123
14. Grode L, Bech BH, Plana-Ripoll O, Bliddal M, Agerholm IE, Humaidan P, Ramlau-Hansen CH (2018) Reproductive life in women with celiac disease; a nationwide, population-based matched cohort study. Hum Reprod 33(8):1538–1547. https://doi.org/10.1093/humrep/dey214
15. Sheiner E, Peleg R, Levy A (2006) Pregnancy outcome of patients with known celiac disease. Eur J Obstet Gynecol Reprod Biol 129:41–45
16. Khashan AS, Henriksen TB, Mortensen PB, McNamee R, McCarthy FP, Pedersen MG, Kenny LC (2010) The impact of maternal celiac disease on birthweight and preterm birth: a Danish population-based cohort study. Hum Reprod 25(2):528–534. https://doi.org/10.1093/humrep/dep409

Chapter 9
Idiopathic Infertility or Unexplained (Unexplained Infertility)

Of the couples who fail to conceive without any identifiable cause, 30% are defined as suffering from "unexplained infertility or idiopathic."

Management depends on the duration of infertility and the age of the female partner. Ray et al. [1] conducted a literature search in the EMBASE, Medline, Ovid, and Cochrane databases using the terms "infertility," "unexplained infertility," "idiopathic infertility," "definition of infertility," "treatment options," "intrauterine insemination," "ovulation induction," "fallopian tube sperm," "GIFT," and "IVF." It seems that there is no uniform definition of the term unexplained infertility. This varies in the literature depending on the duration of infertility and the age of the female partner. The treatment of unexplained infertility is empirical and several items have been hypothesized: wait-and-see management, ovulation stimulation with clomiphene citrate, gonadotropins and aromatase inhibitors, the fallopian tube sperm perfusion, tubal lavage, intrauterine insemination, gamete transfer within the fallopian tubes, and in vitro fertilization.

The standard protocol involves moving from low-tech treatment options to high-tech treatment options. This demonstrates a clear need for multicenter randomized and controlled studies to identify the best treatment option in unexplained infertility using a standard definition.

9.1 Drugs and Idiopathic Infertility

The first approach to the treatment of idiopathic infertility and not due to female factors is generally the use of drugs that stimulate ovocyte production. It is believed that empirical ovarian stimulation favors pregnancy by increasing the number of ovulated eggs and possibly improving implantation, placentation or both through hormonal effects on the endometrium [2]. However, empirical ovarian stimulation (with clomiphene or particularly with gonadotropin) is often complicated by

E. V. Longhi, *Framing Sexual Dysfunctions and Diseases during Fertility Treatment*, https://doi.org/10.1007/978-3-031-76726-5_9

ovarian hyperstimulation syndrome and multiple pregnancies, with an increased risk of preterm birth and associated neonatal morbidity and costs [3]. Recent studies have found that aromatase inhibitors, including letrozole, may be safe and useful agents for ovulation induction in patients with unexplained infertility [4].

Letrozole has been used for ovarian stimulation by fertility specialists since 2001 because it shows fewer side effects compared to clomiphene citrate and fewer chances of multiple pregnancies. A detailed follow-up study on ovulation induction found that letrozole, when compared to a control group of clomiphene, presented significantly lower congenital malformations and chromosomal abnormalities, with an overall rate of 2.4% (1.2% major malformations) compared to clomiphene 4.8% (3.0% major malformations) [5]. Despite this, India banned the use of letrozole in 2011, citing potential risks to newborns [6].

Diamond et al. [7] recruited couples with idiopathic infertility in a multicenter randomized study. The partners were aged between 18 and 40 years with at least one functional fallopian tube and were subjected to ovarian stimulation (up to four cycles) with gonadotropin (301 women), clomiphene (300), or letrozole (299).

After treatment with gonadotropin, clomiphene, or letrozole, clinical pregnancies occurred in 35.5%, 28.3%, and 22.4% of cycles and live births, respectively, in 32.2%, 23.3%, and 18.7%; the pregnancy rates with letrozole were significantly lower than the rates with standard therapy or with gonadotropin alone, but not with clomiphene alone. Among pregnancies with fetal cardiac activity, the rate of multiple gestations with letrozole (9 out of 67 pregnancies, 13%) did not differ significantly from the rate with gonadotropin or clomiphene (42 out of 192, 22%) or clomiphene alone (8 out of 85, 9%), but was lower than the rate with gonadotropin alone (34 out of 107, 32%). All multiple gestations in the clomiphene and letrozole groups were twins, while treatment with gonadotropin produced 24 twin gestations and 10 triplets. At what emotional cost?

From a clinical point of view, unexplained infertility has gone from a diagnosis full of uncertainty and despair to one that, if treated properly, has a positive outlook. But can conceptions soothe the sense of inadequacy, frustration and somatic and psychic diversity compared to other mothers? How can one accept that an unsuspected psychological cause can create this fracture between couples with idiopathic infertility and the rest of the social network?

Unexplained infertility accounts for 22–28% of all infertile couples. The prognosis for a spontaneous pregnancy in such couples is better than those diagnosed with physiological causes of infertility. For these couples, access to psychosexual therapists is often excluded, because specialists believe in a higher chance of success.

The study by Marrero and Ory [8] has shown how unexplained infertility appears to be a nebulous diagnosis that is justified only after a thorough and meticulous investigation of both partners. Even if the five fundamental tests that constitute the infertility investigation reveal no anomaly, there could still be a specific cause. In such couples, spontaneous pregnancies have been reported, with an average cumulative gestation rate of 60% after 3 years [9]. Equating idiopathic infertility with psychogenic infertility is not justified. A definition of psychogenic infertility according to German guidelines is presented. For many women, the effect of infertility and especially medical therapy constitutes a significant emotional stress as they are "healthy and sick" at the same time. Healthy because no physiological causes of infertility are evident, sick because they are infertile without a tangible reason [10].

9.2 The Medical Journeys of Idiopathic Infertility

For this reason, many couples seek solutions in other countries, with the hope that, as unknowns, the couples can receive less critical and disabling treatment. Medical tourism commonly refers to the act of traveling to a foreign country to seek healthcare services [11].

Until recently, the concept of medical tourism was relatively unknown, but the rate of tourism for clinical purposes has seen a sharp acceleration in the last two decades [11]. Modern medical tourism is characterized by an influx of middle-class patients from industrialized countries and wealthy patients from less economically developed countries who utilize the medical services available in foreign destinations. Although medical tourism is a successful economic venture for many countries, exact data regarding the size of the market and revenues remain largely unavailable [12]. According to the medical tourism guide Patients Beyond Borders, in 2015, about 14 million medical travelers went abroad for treatment; as such, it was estimated that the medical tourism market was worth 45.5–72 billion dollars [13]. Another source reported that in 2005 over 19 million trips were made for the purpose of medical tourism for a total value of 20 billion dollars, equivalent to 2.5% of the total volume of annual tourism. It is estimated that this figure will increase to reach 40 million trips per year, a calculated 4% of the total annual volume of medical tourism by 2015 and 6% by 2026 [14].

9.3 Sleep and Idiopathic Infertility

It is well known that the normal biology of fertility is linked to sleep and circadian biology, suggesting that disturbed sleep could have a negative impact on fertility. In fact, several studies have already demonstrated links between sleep disorders, such as the association between obstructive sleep apnea (OSA) and shift work with reproductive dysfunctions. Given that sleep disorders are common and their prevalence seems to be increasing [15], there are good reasons to suggest that they play an important role in the aforementioned decline in population fertility rates. However, despite some understanding of the relationship between sleep disorders, male sexual function, and gonadal hormone secretion, to date there has been a scarcity of research examining the impact of sleep disorders on male fertility. In any case, at the moment, the only therapeutic option available for men suffering from idiopathic infertility is to bypass the identified spermatic anomaly through assisted reproduction technology. The demonstration of a causal link between sleep disorders and idiopathic male infertility has the potential to have a significant impact on the management of infertile couples by providing an additional treatment option for selected individuals.

The study by Matsumoto and Chin [16] revealed that the prevalence of sleep breathing disorders was 24.0–83.8% in males and 9.0–76.6% in females. Since sleep–wake disorders affect homeostasis and metabolic disorders are at the basis of the onset of sleep disorders, the impact of these clinical situations appears significant. Even sex hormones, including progesterone, androgens, and estrogens, are related to respiratory disorders.

In addition, men are more likely to have obstructive sleep apnea syndrome (OSAS), although women are more likely to develop it after menopause. Women generally sleep better than men [17]. They have deeper sleep and a slower age-related decrease in delta activity, a sign of deep sleep. Only 26% of women report an excellent or very good sleep quality. Women with idiopathic infertility over 40 years old are more likely to have sleep disorders. As early as the age of 20 (up to 70 years old), 50% of women develop OSAS. A total of 20% of women have moderate night apnea and 6% develop severe cases [17].

Male rats subjected to intermittent and chronic hypoxia have altered testicular morphology and lose sperm cells during the spermatogenic cycle [18]. It has also been shown that OSAS during childhood affects normal growth and development, compromising the secretion of growth hormone [19]. The data showing an increase in cortisol and adrenocorticotropic hormone levels associated with the interruption of the sleep–wake cycle reflect the effort to maintain wakefulness and possible difficult fertility [20].

9.4 Conclusions

It is not difficult to hypothesize that among medical tourists there are "idiopathic and non-idiopathic infertile" couples, looking for a positive future and unconventional privacy. The escape to foreign countries is for many couples a trip away from reality, from the demands of family, friends, and work colleagues. It is better to disguise a trip as a vacation than to accept having to move elsewhere "to start a new life." It is a pity that twin or multiple births give away the problem: the social and family prejudice that if a multiple birth is obtained, it is most of the time, the result of science, leads many couples to justify themselves with half-truths. "In my family lineage there have been twin births," "We too were surprised…when we had resigned ourselves just being a couple…here is the surprise…we could hardly believe it either… " "Hormonal treatments had nothing to do with the pregnancy…. but after a year…here we are parents. Who would have thought it?" The problems of managing multiple newborns do not elude anxiety or sadness in idiopathic couples. They are often not shared in the couple and too rarely obstetricians and pediatricians advise these couples on a psychological path, where privacy is absolutely guaranteed to feel more complicit in the quality of life and in sexuality. A sexuality, which did not lead to a child, but which can be traced through play and a new lightness of life.

References

1. Ray A, Shah A, Gudi A, Homburg R (2024) Unexplained infertility: an update and review of practice. Reprod Biomed Online 6:591–602. https://doi.org/10.1016/j.rbmo.2012.02.021. Epub 2012 Mar 7. PMID: 22503948
2. Ghesquiere SL, Castelain EG, Spiessens C, Meuleman CL, D'Hooghe TM (2007) Relationship between follicle number and (multiple) live birth rate after controlled ovarian hyperstimulation and intrauterine insemination. Am J Obstet Gynecol 197(6):589.e1–589.e5. https://doi.org/10.1016/j.ajog.2007.05.016
3. Kulkarni AD, Jamieson DJ, Jones HW Jr, Kissin DM, Gallo MF, Macaluso M, Adashi EY (2013) Fertility treatments and multiple births in the United States. N Engl J Med 369:2218–2225. https://doi.org/10.1056/NEJMoa1301467
4. Pavone ME, Bulun SE (2013) Clinical review: the use of aromatase inhibitors for ovulation induction and the superovulation. J Clin Endocrinol Metab 98(5):1838–1844. https://doi.org/10.1210/jc.2013-1328
5. Tulandi T, Martin J, Al-Fadhli R (2006) Congenital malformations among 911 newborns conceived after infertility treatment with letrozole or clomiphene citrate. Fertil Sterile 85(6):1761–1765. https://doi.org/10.1016/j.fertnstert.2006.03.014
6. Sinha K (2011). Finally, an expert group bans the fertility drug Letrozole. The Times of India. October 18. http://timesofindia.indiatimes.com/india/Finally-expert-panel-bans-fertility-drug-Letrozole/articleshow/10395119.cms. Retrieved on 27 Sept 2015
7. Diamond MP, Legro RS, Coutifaris C, Alvero R, Robinson RD, Casson P, Christman GM, Ager J, Huang H, Hansen KR, Baker V, Usadi R, Seungdamrong A, Bates GW, Rosen RM, Haisenleder D, Krawetz SA, Barnhart K, Trussell JC, Ohl D, Jin Y, Santoro N, Eisenberg E, Zhang H, NICHD Reproductive Medicine Network (2015) Letrozole, gonadotropin, or clomiphene for unexplained infertility. N Engl J Med 373(13):1230–1240. https://doi.org/10.1056/NEJMoa1414827
8. Marrero MA, Ory SJ (1991) Unexplained infertility. Curr Opin Obstet Gynecol 3(2):211–218. PMID: 1912353
9. Lobo RA (1993) Unexplained infertility. J Reprod Med 38(4):241–249
10. Wischmann TH (2003) Psychogenic infertility—myths and facts. J Assist Reprod Genet 20(12):485–494. https://doi.org/10.1023/b:jarg.0000013648.74404.9d
11. Debata BR, Patnaik B, Mahapatra SS, Sreekumar K (2013) Measuring efficiency among medical tourism service providers in India. Int J Responsible Tourism 1:24–31
12. Wongkit M, McKercher B (2016) Desired attributes of medical care and medical service providers: a case study of medical tourism in Thailand. J Travel Tour Mark 33:14–27. https://doi.org/10.1080/10548408.2015.1024911
13. Patients Beyond Borders. Medical tourism statistics and facts. [Accessed: November 2016]. From: www.patientsbeyondborders.com/medical-tourism-statistics-facts
14. Guiry M, Scott JJ, Vequist DG (2013) 4th service quality expectations of experienced and potential medical tourists. Int J Health Care Qual Assur 26:433–446. https://doi.org/10.1108/IJHCQA-05-2011-0034
15. Palnitkar G, Phillips CL, Hoyos CM, Marren AJ, Bowman MC, Yee BJ (2018) Linking sleep disturbance to idiopathic male infertility. Sleep Med Rev 42:149–159. https://doi.org/10.1016/j.smrv.2018.07.006

16. Matsumoto T, Chin K (2019) Prevalence of sleep disturbances: sleep disordered breathing, short sleep duration, and non-restorative sleep. Respir Investig 57:227–237. https://doi.org/10.1016/j.resinv.2019.01.008
17. Cojocaru C, Cojocaru E, Pohaci-Antonesei LS, Pohaci-Antonesei CA, Dumitrache-Rujinski S (2023) Sleep apnea syndrome associated with gonadal hormone imbalance (Review). Biomed Rep 19(6):101. https://doi.org/10.3892/br.2023.1683
18. Franklin KA, Sahlin C, Stenlund H, Lindberg E (2018) Sleep apnea is a common event in women. Eur Respir J 41:610–615. https://doi.org/10.1183/09031936.00212711
19. Nieminen P, Löppönen T, Tolonen U, Lanning P, Knip M, Löppönen H (2002) Growth and biochemical markers of growth in children with snoring and obstructive sleep apnea. Pediatrics 109:e55. https://doi.org/10.1542/peds.109.4.e55
20. Nicolaides NC, Vgontzas AN, Kritikou I, Chrousos G (2020) HPA axis and sleep. In: Feingold KR, Anawalt B, Blackman MR et al (eds) Endotext [Internet]. MDText.com, Inc, South Dartmouth

Chapter 10
Couples, Infertility, and the Cost of His Failure

Reduced male fertility contributes to at least 50% of cases of couple infertility. Azoospermia is found in 1–2% of the male population. In the diagnostic process, genetic, endocrine, and lifestyle factors can be considered.

Sperm can be surgically retrieved in many cases of azoospermia, aspermia, and difficult cases of retrograde ejaculation. Such sperm can be used for injection into the oocytes of female partners by intracytoplasmic sperm injection. Treatment with follicle-stimulating hormone is only indicated in hypogonadotropic hypogonadism [1].

But there is more.

The introduction of intracytoplasmic sperm injection (ICSI) into the spectrum of assisted reproduction technologies has offered men suffering from severe disorders of spermatogenesis and azoospermia the opportunity to become fathers.

Various surgical techniques can be used to extract the sperm of these patients from the epididymis and/or the testicle. The surgical recovery of sperm offers a treatment for patients with testicular and/or obstructive azoospermia in cases where microsurgical refertilization is not an option or has already failed.

Among the surgical techniques explored over the years, microsurgical aspiration of sperm from the epididymis (MESA) and testicular sperm extraction (TESE) have become the most popular.

Percutaneous techniques (such as TEFNA) are available but have disadvantages compared to open surgical procedures. Together with the cryopreservation of extracted sperm, these techniques facilitate the recovery of sperm for several attempts at ICSI through a single surgical intervention [2].

Intracytoplasmic sperm injection (ICSI) has revolutionized the treatment of male infertility by allowing men (whose infertility was previously considered uncorrectable) to generate biological offspring.

As a result, surgical sperm recovery for assisted reproduction has developed to support this therapy. Microsurgical techniques have been applied to identify areas of active spermatogenesis within the testicle or to aspirate fluids or tissues containing

E. V. Longhi, *Framing Sexual Dysfunctions and Diseases during Fertility Treatment*, https://doi.org/10.1007/978-3-031-76726-5_10

sperm. The combination of these techniques with in vitro fertilization (IVF)/ICSI has proven to be a powerful approach to the treatment of azoospermic men. The availability of sperm cryopreservation offers a further advantage, eliminating the need to synchronize sperm recovery and ovulation [3].

10.1 But What Does He Think?

It is true that if we interviewed these patients from a psychosexual point of view, they would reveal: guilt for forcing their partner to undergo hormonal therapies, which carry the risk of affecting the woman's health; ejaculation disorders at least 1–2 years before deciding on a surgical therapy for infertility; absent or emotionally unavailable behaviors of the partner in daily life; obsessive thoughts of the patient in the case of fertilization failure and a certain end to the marriage (fear of separation); anhedonia toward sexuality in general, socialization, the network of relatives and friends; feelings of inadequacy with regard to the partner, to their own body, and in comparison with other men; sleep disorders, frequent mistakes at work and low physical energy in the sports practiced [4].

These statements from male patients should be compared with clinical results and success rates.

For example, the study by Nudell et al. [5] recruited 26 patients with obstructive azoospermia to undergo sperm retrieval from the epididymis through a 1 cm incision with local anesthesia and provide sperm for concurrent in vitro fertilization cycles.

The quality of the retrieved sperm, the amount of cryopreserved sperm, as well as the need for anesthesia and the recovery time were evaluated. Fresh epididymal sperm was retrieved in 25 out of 26 patients (96%). In one patient, testicular sperm extraction was necessary. Excess motile sperm were cryopreserved in 24 out of 26 patients (92%); an average total motile count of 4.8 × 10 [6] motile sperm was accumulated. The procedure was performed with 62% of patients receiving minimal intravenous sedation. Post-procedure recovery was quick, with an average return to work time of 2.0 days with an average of 2.0 painkillers taken. Satisfaction with the procedure was high.

Alongside this medical enthusiasm, there are often Her expectations and His anxiety about the outcome. But when are these feelings reported? To whom? When are they evaluated during an infertility journey?

Often only following a parental failure, are couples referred to a sexologist.

A case: a couple, respectively, 38 years old (He, mechanic) and 32 years old (She, executive secretary), arrives at the consultation anxious, distant, argumentative and with feelings of anxiety, depression, and anger. They state that the partner, azoospermic, had turned to an andrologist, initially concerning erectile dysfunction, about 2 years before. During the clinical investigations, azoospermia is also diagnosed. He is informed of the surgical technique for infertility, but depression takes over and only after 6 months does he return to the andrologist to review the situation. In the meantime, the partner shows disinterest in sexuality, but with the birth of children by her sister and some work colleagues, she encourages her partner to consider an infertility journey.

They start the process with little conviction and above all with the fear of experiencing too much physical pain and not being able to have a sexual life. They close in on themselves: they see their friends less and less, they keep the secret from everyone. The partner undergoes hormonal stimulation and in vitro fertilization twice. Two failures. They think there is nothing more to do, but for them it is difficult to accept the situation. They try a third time, the last. The partner is urgently hospitalized for an ectopic pregnancy. The husband thinks not only that if he lost his wife it would certainly be "his fault alone" but also that she would do well to divorce Him.

The partner recovers physically in a relatively short time, but cohabitation becomes increasingly difficult. The arguments increase exponentially and sexuality is completely forgotten. The couple enjoys a strong emotional bond and because of this they turn again to the andrologist for advice. Hence the referral to the sexologist.

Now the couple has decided to accept a family of two, but the journey was not without suffering. They enjoy (report) a satisfying sexuality, but the secret of their failed experience still prevails.

But there is more.

Some studies [6] have evaluated how much advanced paternal age can influence the outcome of intracytoplasmic sperm injection (ICSI) (following the cryopreservation of sperm obtained through testicular sperm extraction (TESE)).

10.2 Question of Paternal Age

The review by Kidd et al. [7] concluded that the advanced age of the male partner is associated with a lower sperm volume, and an inferior sperm motility and morphology, but no change in sperm concentration was noted. This review found that advanced male age can negatively affect fertility, particularly in men over the age of 50. Recently, some studies have also evaluated the effect of paternal age on sperm characteristics and found similar decreases in total sperm count in the total count of mobile sperm and in total sperm volume.

In this particular case, it was a 14-year study that began in 1997. All participating patients had undergone a complete physical examination of the genitals to assess the anatomy of the seminal vesicles, the prostate, the distal vas deferens. and the ejaculatory ducts. Male patients diagnosed with azoospermia underwent TESE with routine cryopreservation. The thawed testicular sperm were subsequently used for a total of 212 cycles of ICSI until August 2010 [7]. Male partners were stratified into age categories at 5-year intervals (31–35 years, 36–40 years, and > 40–51 years).

As many studies have suggested, advanced male age is correlated with the risk of chromosomal abnormalities in sperm and could increase the rate of miscarriages [8].

It is understandable that such an event would mortify both members of the couple and, especially, generate a sense of guilt on the male side. The unexpected outcome of a fertility nipped in the bud, with a miscarriage of hers, openly manifests the inadequacy of the partner, remorse for having been the cause of a life nipped in the bud.

It is difficult for these couples to overcome infertility, failure, miscarriage, and a life perspective for two. The male sexual dysfunctions that arise after similar experiences are a clear attestation, on the part of the partner, of absolute responsibility and condemnation. A way to protect the partner and make her alien to failure.

But that is not all.

Some studies have shown that substance abuse is correlated with mental health problems, especially in infertile men. For example, the use of cannabis often precedes depression and suicidal behavior [9]. The persistent use of more substances is particularly higher in men after a procreative failure [10]. Depressed people are at a higher risk of suicide when they abuse substances [11], such as early use of marijuana, alcohol, and other illicit drugs [12]. However, the relationship between substance use and depression in infertile couples remains unknown.

10.3 Underlying Diseases and Obesity

Despite advances in understanding male infertility, the *idiopathic* anomalies of sperm still represent about 30% of male infertility. However, it has been found that a variety of medical conditions affect sperm parameters, such as kidney diseases, liver failure, hemochromatosis, chronic obstructive pulmonary disease, cystic fibrosis, and multiple sclerosis [13].

An Italian study on 2100 infertile men examined the relationship between the Charlson comorbidity index (CCI), seminal parameters, and hormonal levels. The study [14] showed that, with an increase in the CCI (an indicator of poor health), the sperm parameters deteriorate and the levels of the follicle-stimulating hormone (FSH) increase, suggesting a pituitary compensation in the context of spermatogenic dysfunction.

The mechanism through which medical conditions can have an impact on fertility includes effects on hormonal levels, impairment of sexual function (including ejaculatory function), or impairment of testicular/spermatogenesis function. By medically optimizing the man's health, the improvement of the pathological state can improve sperm parameters [15], sexual function, and fertility potential.

Not to forget that obesity is associated with male infertility, probably due to hormonal changes secondary to excess adipose tissue.

In a multi-institutional retrospective cohort study, Bieniek et al. [16] demonstrated an inverse relationship between body mass index (BMI) and testosterone, testosterone/estradiol ratio, ejaculate volume, sperm concentration, and morphology.

The authors also reported higher rates of azoospermia and oligospermia among obese men (respectively 12.7% and 31.7%) compared to normal weight men (9.8% and 24.5%).

Furthermore, couples composed of an overweight or obese man [17] with a female partner of normal BMI had a longer conception time compared to couples with normal weight male partners.

Couples undergoing assisted reproduction technology (ART), where the male partner is obese [18], have also recorded a decrease in pregnancy rates and an increase in pregnancy interruptions, probably due to higher rates of DNA fragmentation in obese men.

10.4 Urogenital Diseases and Infertility

Men with congenital genitourinary defects (GU), such as cryptorchidism, hypospadias, and anomalies of the male external genitals, may have a spermatogenic insufficiency caused by the genetic defects underlying these conditions. In particular, these patients may have significant associated phenotypes.

The study by Schneuer et al. [19] is significant: male genital anomalies, hypospadias, and retained testicles have been linked to adult male reproductive disorders, testicular cancer, and decreased fertility.

Between 1970 and 1999, 350,835 boys born in Western Australia were recruited and followed up until 2016 through the linkage of data to register for hospital admissions, congenital anomalies, cancer. and assisted reproduction technologies (ART). The study factors were hypospadias or retained testicles, while the study outcomes were testicular cancer, paternity, and the use of antiretroviral therapy for male infertility.

Among the 350,835 boys, 2484 (0.7%) were diagnosed with hypospadias and 7499 (2.1%) with retained testicles. There were 505 (0.1%) cases of testicular cancer: 109,471 (31.2%) patients had children and 2682 (0.8%) had undergone fertility treatment with ART. Testicle retention was associated with a more than twofold increase in the risk of testicular cancer and hypospadias with an increase of almost 40%, although this increase was not significant.

Both hypospadias and retained testicles were associated with a 21% reduction in paternity. Testicular retention was associated with a twofold increase in the use of antiretroviral therapy. For every 6 months of delay in orchidopexy, there was a 6% increase in the risk of testicular cancer, a 5% increase in the risk of future use of ART, and a 1% reduction in paternity.

10.5 Conclusions

In conclusion, male reproductive failure shows that being underweight, overweight, or obese, or having urogenital diseases, even during childhood and adolescence, is associated with negative health consequences throughout life.

Underweight among children and adolescents is associated with a higher risk of infectious diseases and, for girls of childbearing age, is associated with adverse pregnancy outcomes, including maternal mortality, complications of childbirth, preterm birth, and intrauterine growth retardation.

Overweight during childhood and adolescence is associated with a higher risk of chronic disorders such as type 2 diabetes.

However, the greater weight concerns the couple's relationship, the joint planning, the quality of sexual life, the minimal percentages of procreative success for the male part, even with the recourse to surgery.

When the cause of infertility and lack of parenthood is of male origin, the understanding and cooperation of the partner do not seem sufficient to overcome the physical, mental, and social consequences. The partner will sooner or later present depression, dissatisfaction, and revenge toward the partner and his family, as the original source of inadequacy and unhappiness.

The psychosexual therapist in these cases can desensitize the aggression, the revenge, and the consequent resentment in the relationship of the couple.

Even more so, the initial care of an infertile patient and his partner can be a valuable contribution for the couple and the medical team to share a double procreative project, whether in the case of success or failure. As to prevent conditions of food, alcohol, and substance dependence in subsequent follow-ups or the absence of intimacy.

References

1. Fedder J, Carlsen E, Jørgensen N, CFS J (2021) Treatment of male infertility. Ugeskr Laeger 183(48):V05210402. Danish. PMID: 34852902
2. Diemer T, Hauptmann A, Weidner W (2010) Therapie der Azoospermie. Urologe 50:38–46. https://doi.org/10.1007/s00120-010-2442-1
3. Ald M, Niederberger CS, Ross LS (2004) Surgical sperm retrieval for assisted reproduction. Minerva Ginecol 56(3):217–222. PMID: 15258533
4. Longhi EV. Pilot study on the course of fertility surgery in a group of infertile men (54 azoospermic, 22 with ejaculation disorder) in progress since 2022 at the Center for Sexual Medicine, IRCCS San Raffaele, Vita & Salute University, Milan, Italy: preview of partial data
5. Nudell DM, Conaghan J, Pedersen RA, Givens CR, Schriock ED, Turek PJ (1998) The mini-micro-epididymal sperm aspiration for sperm retrieval: a study of urological outcomes. Hum Reprod 13(5):1260–1265. https://doi.org/10.1093/humrep/13.5.1260. PMID: 9647557
6. Tsai YR, Lan KC, Kung FT, Lin PY, Chiang HJ, Lin YJ, Huang FJ (2013) The effect of advanced paternal age on the outcomes of assisted reproductive techniques among patients with azoospermia using cryopreserved testicular spermatozoa. Taiwan J Obstet Gynecol 52(3):351–355

7. Kidd SA, Eskenazi B, Wyrobek AJ (2001) Effects of male age on semen quality and fertility: a review of the literature. Fertil Steril 75:237–248
8. Sloter E, Nath J, Eskenazi B, Wyrobek AJ (2004) Effects of male age on the frequencies of germinal chromosomal anomalies and hereditary in humans and rodents. Fertil Steril 81:925–943
9. Halladay JE, MacKillop J, Munn C, Jack SM, Georgiades K (2020) Use of cannabis as a risk factor for depression, anxiety and suicide: epidemiological associations and implications for nurses. J Addict Nurses 31:92–101. https://doi.org/10.1097/JAN.0000000000000334
10. Williams GC, Patte KA, Ferro MA, Leatherdale ST (2021) Associations between longitudinal patterns of substance use and symptoms of anxiety and depression in a sample of Canadian high school students. Int J Environ Res Public Health 18:10468. https://doi.org/10.3390/ijerph181910468
11. Murthy P, Mahadevan J, Chand PK (2019) Treatment of substance use disorders with concomitant severe mental health disorders. Curr Opin Psychiatry 32:293–299. https://doi.org/10.1097/YCO.0000000000000510
12. Brook DW, Brook JS, Zhang C, Cohen P, Whiteman M (2002) Drug use and risk of major depressive disorder, alcohol dependence, and substance use disorders. Arch Gen Psychiatry 59:1039–1044. https://doi.org/10.1001/archpsyc.59.11.1039
13. Cavallini G (2006) Male idiopathic oligoasthenoteratozoospermia. Asian J Androl 8(2):143–157. https://doi.org/10.1111/j.1745-7262.2006.00123.x
14. Ventimiglia E, Capogrosso P, Boeri L et al (2015) Infertility as an indicator of men's overall health: results of a cross-sectional survey. Fertil Sterile 104(1):48–55. https://doi.org/10.1016/j.fertnstert.2015.04.020
15. Lotti F, Maggi M (2018) Sexual dysfunctions and male infertility. Nat Rev Urol 15(5):287–307. https://doi.org/10.1038/nrurol.2018.20
16. Bieniek JM, Kashanian JA, Deibert CM et al (2016) Influence of increased body mass index on sperm and reproductive hormonal parameters in a multi-institutional cohort of subfertile men. Fertil Sterile 106(5):1070–1075. https://doi.org/10.1016/j.fertnstert.2016.06.041
17. Campbell JM, Lane M, Owens JA, Bakos HW et al (2015) Paternal obesity negatively affects male fertility and assisted reproduction outcomes: a systematic review and meta-analysis. Reprod Biomed Online 31(5):593–604. https://doi.org/10.1016/j.rbmo.2015.07.012
18. Dupont C, Faure C, Sermondade N, Boubaya M, Eustache F, Clément P, Briot P, Berthaut I, Levy V, Cedrin-Durnerin I, Benzacken B, Chavatte-Palmer P, Levy R (2013) Obesity leads to a higher risk of sperm DNA damage in infertile patients. Asian J Androl 15(5):622–625. https://doi.org/10.1038/aja.2013.65
19. Schneuer FJ, Milne E, Jamieson SE, Pereira G, Hansen M, Barker A, Holland AJA, Bower C, Nassar N (2018) Association between male genital anomalies and adult male reproductive disorders: a population-based data linkage study spanning more than 40 years. Lancet Child Adolesc Health 2(10):736–743. https://doi.org/10.1016/S2352-4642(18)30254-2. Epub 2018 Aug 30. PMID: 30236382

Chapter 11
Couples, Infertility, and the Cost of Her Failure

The scientific literature has always investigated the correlation between the duration of infertility and the ability of couples to reinvest emotionally in themselves and their future goals. In practice: How do couples overcome the failures of assisted reproduction treatments and generally of infertility? How do clinicians deal with this eventuality? Do they worry about the couples' emotions?

If we consider that in 2005 alone, 923 clinics in 30 countries carried out 418,111 treatment cycles (IVF (118,074), ICSI (203,329), replacement of frozen embryos (79,140), egg donation (ED, 11,475), preimplantation genetic diagnosis/screening (5846), and in vitro maturation (247)), *we are facing a percentage increase of 13.6% compared to 2004, partly due to the inclusion of 28,417 cycles from Turkey.* European data on intrauterine insemination using the husband/partner's sperm (IUI-H) and a donor's sperm (IUI-D) were reported by 21 countries and included 128,908 IUI-H cycles and 20,568 IUI-D cycles [1].

Furthermore, in 16 countries where all clinics were registered in the IVF registry, 1115 cycles were performed per million inhabitants. For in vitro fertilization, the clinical pregnancy rates for aspiration and transfer were 26.9% and 30.3%, respectively. For intracytoplasmic sperm injection (ICSI), the corresponding rates were 28.5% and 30.9%. After IUI-H, the clinical pregnancy rate was 12.6% per insemination in women <40 years old. After in vitro fertilization and ICSI, the distribution of the transfer of one, two, three, and four or more embryos was 20.0%, 56.1%, 21.5%, and 2.3%, respectively. There are huge differences between countries. The distribution of single, twin, and triplet births after IVF and ICSI was 78.2%, 21.0%, and 0.8%, respectively. This gives a total multiple birth rate of 21.8% compared to 22.7% in 2004 and 23.1% in 2003. In women <40 years old, IUI-H was associated with a rate of twin and triple pregnancies of 11.0% and 1.1%, respectively.

If we only consider these percentages, which are far lower than today's data, it is clear how a failure of such treatments can be a traumatic experience and not always overcome by individuals and the couple. Moreover, for clinicians, a better understanding of how patients' infertility history is linked to their emotional adjustment

E. V. Longhi, *Framing Sexual Dysfunctions and Diseases during Fertility Treatment*, https://doi.org/10.1007/978-3-031-76726-5_11

during treatment, can help fertility health services to identify which patients will experience greater emotional difficulties at the beginning of treatment and will need more support during the clinical process.

But we know that not all centers provide for the figure of the psychosexologist.

The approach to assisted reproduction technology (ART) treatments and generally to infertility appears very medical (it is mostly teams of biologists, geneticists, andrologists, gynecologists, and endocrinologists) and often the couple's story and their sexuality is not examined, because it is considered to have little influence on the couple's desire for parenthood. Or worse, it is taken for granted.

Moreover, the literature in these cases shows contradictory studies.

11.1 Duration of Infertility and Failure

Markestad et al. [2] examined the effect of the number of treatments undergone on psychological distress and found a standard trend of anxiety and depression after a greater number of treatments. Conversely, Slade et al. [3], in a prospective study of 144 couples, found a higher negative mood at the beginning of the first cycle, lower in the second and even higher in the third cycle. Boivin et al. [4] examined the impact of treatment failure on psychological functioning by comparing three groups of women with various levels of treatment failure, controlling for the effect of duration of infertility: patients without previous treatments, patients undergoing first-line conventional treatments, and patients who start in vitro fertilization after unsuccessful first-line treatments. The results indicated that patients undergoing first-line treatments reported the highest level of distress (marital, sexual, personal, and related to infertility) of the three groups.

The authors concluded that the relationship between treatment failure and patient adjustment is independent of time, and that it is the repetitiveness of treatment failure (and not the time spent in treatment or the duration of infertility) that conditions the emotional and relational adjustment of couples.

This leads to the belief that it is not the duration of infertility that discourages couples, but the failure of therapies and the acceptance of the absence of parenthood. It follows that even intimacy in couples loses meaning. If not supported in a sexological journey post failure, they will hardly resume a playful sexual life and a more intense relationship between two, especially when during fertility paths, the couple has experienced clinical experiences that have put the life of the pregnant woman at risk or intergenerational conflicts have emerged.

When studying emotional adjustment to infertility, it is of primary importance to take into consideration the subjective meaning of parenthood and the absence of children in the life of every couple.

11.2 Him, Her, and the Professionals

The study by Greil et al. [5] recruited 22 infertile married couples living in the western part of New York State to highlight the impact of infertility between the two genders.

Results: Wives experienced infertility as a catastrophic failure of role. Husbands tended to see infertility as a disconcerting event but not as a tragedy. Couples in general tended to see infertility as an almost exclusively female problem.

However, frustration and lack of communication were typical consequences of the confrontation between husbands' and wives' perspectives on infertility.

Communication with clinicians appeared no less problematic. These interactions between wives, husbands, and medical professionals could influence the sharing of treatment and lead to ignoring therapeutic options. Not to mention attributing to clinicians, the blame for treating couples as "guinea pigs" and not as people to accompany on a medium-long journey.

Furthermore, in their review on the emotional adaptation of women to ART treatments, Verhaak et al. [6] suggested that the negative emotional responses observed were strongly correlated with the treatment outcome, i.e., the threat of a permanent absence of children. Therefore, the acceptance of the lack of children was identified as an important predictor of the emotional response to treatment [7].

Moreover, evaluating 187 nonpregnant women according to personality traits, stress threshold, coping ability, and social support, the emotional response and vulnerability of these women before the start of each treatment were hypothesized. The results indicated the importance of neuroticism as a vulnerability factor in the emotional response to a severe stress factor, helplessness and marital dissatisfaction as additional risk factors, and social support to monitor levels of anxiety and depression after a failed fertility treatment.

11.3 The Irrationality of Infertility

In a study by Fekkes et al. [8], 425 men and 447 women intending to undergo in vitro fertilization treatment were evaluated with a questionnaire that assessed four areas of health-related quality of life: emotional, physical, cognitive, and social health.

Results: Young men and women (aged between 21 and 30 years) planning in vitro fertilization had more short-term social and emotional problems compared to people of the same age group in the control group. No substantial differences were found in cognitive and physical functioning for all age groups of men and women planning in vitro fertilization compared to the general population. Particularly, widespread irrational parental cognitions emerged among younger women such as "a life without children makes no sense," "without children I am not a woman," and "a couple without children has no future."

Since a longer history of infertility and cumulative failed ART treatments faced infertile couples with the possibility of a permanent absence of children [9], it is undeniable that these factors make the importance of parenthood more salient along the infertility process, often reducing compliance.

The study by Moura-Ramos et al. [10] recruited 70 infertile couples (70 women and 70 men) who completed self-report questionnaires assessing emotional adjustment and infertility stress during the hormonal stimulation phase of an ART cycle.

Results: The number of previous ART cycles and the duration of infertility have differently influenced the adaptation of women and men. Having undergone a greater number of treatment cycles may have confronted men with the increasingly likely prospect of remaining childless, favoring their acceptance and reducing their discomfort, while women saw each new ART cycle as a moment of hope to achieve pregnancy.

11.4 Sleep and Infertility

Sleep disorders can also interfere with women's reproductive processes, such as prolonged conception time, a reduced chance of conception, an increased rate of miscarriage, and a low birth weight of the baby. Therefore, the sleep conditions of women undergoing in vitro fertilization treatment with increased emotional distress should be monitored to improve ART outcomes.

Lin et al. [11] revealed that 23% and 46% of women who had received in vitro fertilization had sleep disorders during the oocyte retrieval and the implantation process, respectively. Goldstein et al. [12] determined that 57%, 43%, and 29% of women who received in vitro fertilization experienced sleep disorders during the pretreatment, stimulation, and post embryo transfer (ET) process, respectively. It was determined that hormones such as the anti-mullerian hormone (AMH), the follicle-stimulating hormone (FSH), and the total basal pretreatment sleep time (TST) can influence the patient's sleep during the oocyte retrieval process.

The Beck Anxiety Inventory and the Beck Depression Inventory are the most used questionnaires in research in addition to the Pittsburgh Sleep Quality Index (PSQI). This self-assessment test determines sleep quality with seven sections. These sections are: (1) subjective sleep quality, (2) sleep latency, (3) sleep duration, (4) sleep efficiency, (5) sleep disturbances, (6) use of sleep medication, and (7) degree of daytime dysfunction. There are a total of 19 questions with scores that can range from 0 to 21. The global sum of "5" is the limit of good sleep quality, while the patient with a score above 5 experiences significant sleep disorders [13].

Emotional distress and sleep disorders could contribute to the success of in vitro fertilization treatment. Therefore, the ovulation induction (hormonal stimulation) period of in vitro fertilization treatment is the critical time to assess the status and association of such psychological distress and sleep quality. However, the literature exploring this issue is scarce.

The study by Lin et al. [11] concluded that the majority of women who received in vitro fertilization treatments were anxious (43%), depressed (30%), and had sleep disorders (43%). Anxiety is particularly linked to sleep disorders. It is suggested that the healthcare professional understands these common problems when assisting women undergoing these complicated reproductive treatments. Tools such as mental health assessment and sleep history can be used to provide a more comprehensive care model.

11.5 Conclusions

It would be a methodological error not to address the "failure" before proceeding with assisted reproduction technology treatments and general infertility. Couples, such as clinicians, often feel uncomfortable and unprepared to face outcomes different from the desire for parenthood.

Although it seems that the partners of women undergoing ART show a faster and more rational acceptance process, the patients, unfulfilled in their desire for motherhood, often also refuse intimacy. Resentment, anguish, and "betrayal" of much spent energy more often lead patients to show conflictual behaviors within the couple and to experience sexuality as superfluous and meaningless.

In these cases, the psychosexologist must review the couple's contract, desensitize the conflict, and bring the relationship back to a level of mutual trust. A very tiring process for those couples who have lost the motivation of their bond and who tend to feel undeserving of serenity and pleasure. In some cases, food addiction compensates for the need to compensate for "an undeserved and unjust defeat." Confidence in the future, in medical teams, in social relationships falls. Clinicians in general should also reflect beyond the medical parameters and promote a more empathetic relationship with patients, at least to satisfy, if not the desire for parenthood, a participatory and welcoming relationship.

References

1. Andersen AN, Goossens V, Bhattacharya S, Ferraretti AP, Kupka MS, de Mouzon J et al (2009) Assisted reproduction technology and intrauterine inseminations in Europe, 2005: results generated from European registries by ESHRE. Hum Reprod 24:1267–1287. https://doi.org/10.1093/humrep/dep035
2. Markestad CL, Montgomery LM, Bartsch RA (1998) Effects of infertility and duration of medical treatment on psychological, marital, and sexual functioning. Int J Rehabil Health 4:233–243. https://doi.org/10.1023/A:1022966829561
3. Slade P, Emery J, Lieberman BA (1997) A prospective and longitudinal study on emotions and relationships in in vitro fertilization treatment. Hum Reprod 12:183–190. https://doi.org/10.1093/humrep/12.1.183

4. Boivin J, Bunting L, Collins JA, Nygren KG (2007) International estimates on the prevalence of infertility and on the demand for treatment: potential need and demand for medical care for infertility. Hum Reprod 22:1506–1512. https://doi.org/10.1093/humrep/dem046
5. Greil AL, Leitko TA, Porter KL (1988) Infertility: him and her. Gend Soc 2:172–199. https://doi.org/10.1177/089124388002002004
6. Verhaak CM, Smeenk JM, Evers AW, Kremer JA, Kraaimaat FW, Braat DD (2007) Women's emotional adjustment to IVF: a systematic review of 25 years of research. Hum Reprod Update 13:27–36. https://doi.org/10.1093/humupd/dml040
7. Verhaak CM, Smeenk JM, Evers AW, van Minnen A, Kremer JA, Kraaimaat FW (2005) Predicting emotional response to unsuccessful fertility treatment: a prospective study. J Behav Med 28:181–190. https://doi.org/10.1007/s10865-005-3667-0
8. Fekkes M, Buitendijk SE, Verrips GHW, Braat DDM, Brewaeys AMA, Dolfing JG et al (2003) Health-related quality of life in relation to gender and age in couples planning IVF treatment. Hum Reprod 18:1536–1543. https://doi.org/10.1093/humrep/deg276
9. Boivin J, Andersson L, Skoog-Svanberg A, Hjelmstedt A, Collins A, Bergh T (1998) Psychological reactions during in-vitro fertilization: similar response pattern in husbands and wives. Hum Reprod 13:3262–3267. https://doi.org/10.1093/humrep/13.11.3262
10. Moura-Ramos M, Gameiro S, Canavarro MC, Soares I, Santos TA (2012) The indirect effect of contextual factors on the emotional distress of infertile couples. Psychol Health 27(5):533–549. https://doi.org/10.1080/08870446.2011.598231. Epub 2011 Jul 19. PMID: 21767233
11. Lin YH, Chueh KH, Lin JL (2016) Somatic symptoms, sleep disturbance and psychological distress among women undergoing oocyte pick-up and in vitro fertilisation-embryo transfer. J Clin Nurs 25(11–12):1748–1756. https://doi.org/10.1111/jocn.13194
12. Goldstein CA, Lanham MS, Smith YR, O'Brien LM (2017) Sleep in women undergoing in vitro fertilization: a pilot study. Sleep Med 32:105–113. https://doi.org/10.1016/j.sleep.2016.12.007
13. Buysse DJ, Reynolds CF, Monk TH, Hoch CC, Yeager AL, Kupfer DJ (1991) Quantification of subjective sleep quality in healthy older men and women using the Pittsburgh Sleep Quality Index (PSQI). Sleep 14(4):331–338. https://doi.org/10.1093/sleep/14.4.331

Chapter 12
Coping with Infertility: Validity of Psychosexual Counseling

Most couples choose coping strategies to deal with infertility and mitigate the resulting mental pressure. Coping strategies are a set of cognitive, emotional, and behavioral efforts to interpret, analyze, and modify a stressful situation [1]. Lazarus et al. define coping as a response to mental pressure such as infertility. Such a reaction is a personal attempt to overcome harmful, threatening, or difficult circumstances [2].

Coping strategies are classified into four groups: active coping, active avoidance, passive avoidance, and meaning-based coping [3].

The effectiveness of any coping strategy depends on the controllable or uncontrollable emotional conditions of the individual and the social and cultural context to which they belong. For example, some coping strategies to deal with maladjustment and psychological problems could have reverse effects in various cultural environments [4]. The study by Aflakseir and Zarei [4] examined the role of coping strategies (active avoidance, passive avoidance, active confrontation, and meaning-based) in predicting infertility stress in a group of women seeking treatment for infertility in Shiraz. One hundred and twenty infertile women were recruited from various infertility clinics in Shiraz: the patients completed the Infertility Problem Stress Inventory and the Ways of Coping Scale (passive avoidance, active avoidance, active confrontation, meaning-based).

The results showed that the participants had the highest scores in passive avoidance coping strategies followed by meaning-based coping, active confrontation coping, and active avoidance coping. The results also indicated that women who used more active avoidance coping strategies reported less infertility stress.

Furthermore, both the close and the global interactions of couples can lead to each spouse being influenced by the choice of coping strategies of their partner and the psychological damage resulting from infertility. A coping strategy adopted by each spouse could also affect the mental health of their partner [5]. The studies by Peterson et al. [5] grouped 1169 Danish women and 1081 Danish men before starting assisted reproduction treatment. To examine the couple as a unit of analysis

E. V. Longhi, *Framing Sexual Dysfunctions and Diseases during Fertility Treatment*, https://doi.org/10.1007/978-3-031-76726-5_12

questionnaires using the actor–partner interdependence model and a follow-up analysis of variance were used.

The partner's use of active avoidance coping was correlated with an increase in personal, marital, and social distress for both men and women. Women's use of active coping strategies was correlated with an increase in male marital distress, while the partner's use of meaning-based coping was associated with a decrease in marital distress in men and an increase in social distress in women.

The existing coping strategies mainly focus on the individual. However, coping strategies that can reduce an individual's infertility stress can also negatively affect the mental health of the partner. Therefore, considering the interactive effect of couples' coping strategies, it is essential to identify coping strategies whose resulting interactive effect is accompanied by a reduction in the psychological burden of infertility in both men and women, particularly in situations where men and women do not behave in the same way to bear the psychological and social burden of infertility. In traditional societies where infertility is mainly attributed to women, they are more vulnerable to the social stigma of infertility compared to men.

The study by Kaya and Oskay [6] was conducted on 278 infertile women who applied for treatment between December 2017 and April 2018 at the Department of Reproductive Medicine, Endocrinology and Infertility of Istanbul University Hospital. The data were collected using the Infertility Stigmatization Scale (ISS), the Beck Hopelessness Scale (BHS), and the COPE Inventory (COPE). *Results*: It was found that infertile women experienced mild stigmatization and minimal despair. In many cultures, failed pregnancy and the absence of parenthood are perceived as a reproductive failure that mostly leads to social stigma. Infertile women also experience negative feelings such as anxiety, depression, and despair, which makes ways to cope with infertility significant for a sense of stability. It was established that infertile women mainly used a religious coping strategy to stabilize emotions.

12.1 Counseling Strategies

In an attempt to provide psychological support to infertile couples, Zurlo et al. developed a model (7) of predictive variables of mental health in infertile couples undergoing treatment that demonstrates the importance of adaptive coping strategies for the mental health of infertile couples.

The effect of some counseling methods on the coping strategies of couples undergoing assisted reproduction techniques was also evaluated.

A total of 254 infertile couples were recruited and completed a questionnaire composed of sociodemographic, Fertility Problem Inventory-Short Form (FPI-SF), Coping Orientation to Problem Experienced-New Italian Version (COPE-NIV), and State-Trait Anxiety Inventory-Y (STAI-Y).

The results revealed that social concern and couple relational concern, in both partners, and the need for parenthood, in female partners, had positive correlations with anxiety and depression. Furthermore:

1. Seeking social support and avoidant coping were correlated with increasing levels of anxiety in both partners, while positive attitude coping strategies were correlated with lower levels of anxiety in female partners.
2. Problem-solving and avoidant coping played a moderating role between specific dimensions of infertility-related stress and anxiety.
3. Problem-solving exacerbated the negative effects of social concern, while avoidant coping buffered the negative effects of various dimensions of infertility-related stress in both partners.

Interventions to improve stress management and psychological health in infertile couples should consider that the adequacy of coping strategies is intrinsically specific to the situation. Therefore, it follows that patient-centered clinical interventions should consider the potential inadequacy of individuals, problem-solving strategies, and even the instinct of denial and avoidance of the infertility problem could be an effective strategy for some couples to cope with the stress related to infertility.

One study evaluated the effect of the positive adjustment intervention of coping using a smartphone to provide psychological support to women undergoing treatment for infertility and found that the program was associated with a reduction in the psychological burden of women during treatment [8]. Furthermore, the positive effect of cognitive-behavioral interventions on reducing stress in women undergoing assisted reproduction technologies was reported [9].

These findings suggest that adaptive coping strategies can reduce the psychological burden of infertility. Therefore, it is necessary for couple strategies to focus on the interaction between couples in order to reduce the psychological burden resulting from infertility and treatment in couples undergoing treatment.

12.2 The Psychosexual Intervention

When the desire for a child is particularly difficult to realize due to infertility, the ability to manage stress and frustration is severely tested. In these circumstances, family and friends are of great help, but their influence could create additional expectations that the couple cannot succumb to. Consider a couple where one of the members is an adopted child, or a man in his second marriage who fears losing his younger partner in the absence of parenthood, or a mixed culture couple where traditions require parenthood to give value to the couple.

The couple's history, therefore, would appear to be the first element to start from to identify feelings that would be useful in planning a journey together or reflecting on alternative solutions to assisted reproductive technology.

This view of reality allows one to act on facts and interact with people in a way that is more congruent with one's own needs and desires. However, it requires a reality check in which thoughts and emotions become explicit and recognized, as much as possible, so as not to superimpose them on reality, generating confusion. Why the psychosexual therapist?

Because this figure also examines the sexual history of individuals and the couple's style, hypothesizes their potential as adults even after possible parenthood. Often sexuality and fertility are associated in a single process by patients and the couple inevitably falls short.

You cannot be parents if you are not an adult couple first.

But there is more.

The discomfort caused by infertility produces a feeling of low motivation for the future, of failure, due to an inadequate, unsuitable, unreliable body compared to fertile bodies. It is a real identity crisis, with a loss of value of one's role in the society, in the profession, in the couple, and in the families of origin.

Three are three types of counseling used so far:

- *European Society of Human Reproduction and Embryology (ESHRE) implications counseling or decision-making counseling.* The fundamental purpose is to allow subjects to understand and reflect during the treatment proposal on the implications that this could have for them, for their families, and for any children. This type of consultation should be available before each treatment.
- *Support counseling, defined by international literature and by ESHRE support counseling.* The aim is to accompany couples in times of stress and difficulty, e.g., couples who cannot access therapies (due to worsening underlying diseases), couples who show difficulty in undertaking the treatment recommended by clinicians, and couples who have to face the failure of a treatment cycle.
- *Therapeutic counseling so defined by international literature and by ESHRE.* The aim is to assist couples in making them aware of their own infertility, the partner's infertility, and the possible failure of the clinical treatment.

An Italian study by Valoriani et al. [10] has evaluated in depth the emotional state of patients admitted for the first visit. Specifically, they investigated the emotional state of the two members of an infertile couple, also considering their biomedical and sociodemographic characteristics. A total of 309 couples who had presented for the first visit at the Infertility Unit were evaluated by a multidisciplinary team in relation to their infertility. The multidisciplinary team was composed of a gynecologist, an andrologist, and a clinical psychologist. Two standardized tools were administered by the clinical psychologist to the two members of the couple: the Edinburgh Depression Scale (EDS) and the General Health Questionnaire-Form 12 (GHQ-12), for screening of mood disorder, particularly depression and anxiety. They found a positive response for 62% of couples and from this data it can be inferred that starting from the first interview for ART, the couples experience deep emotional stress that cannot be ignored.

Similarly, the study by Reis et al. [11] investigated the psychological impact of couples undergoing single and multiple cycles of assisted reproduction.

In this prospective research at the Medically Assisted Reproduction Unit of the Centro Hospitalar de São João, Porto, Portugal, 89 couples with a diagnosis of infertility were divided into two groups:

1. couples who had started ART for the first time (43) and,
2. couples who had pursued ART repeatedly (46).

The participants completed the Beck Depression Inventory-II (BDI-II) and the State-Trait Anxiety Inventory-Form Y (STAI-Y) before the first or subsequent treatment cycle.

Results: Couples who were undergoing ART for the first time showed higher levels of anxiety compared to couples who were practicing ART repeatedly ($p < 0.05$). Depression levels appeared higher in couples who were experiencing repeated ART ($p < 0.05$). In both study groups, women and men showed higher levels of state anxiety compared to trait anxiety ($p < 0.05$). Regarding depression, there are significant differences between the sexes in both groups, showing higher values in women compared to men ($p < 0.01$).

But there is more.

The difficulties in psychological adaptation to the diagnosis of infertility and treatments with assisted reproduction technology (ART) have shown an influence on sperm quality. The biological and psychological aspects of infertility seem not to be independent [12].

The cross-sectional study by Bártolo et al. [12] conducted at the Medically Assisted Reproduction Unit of the Centro Hospitalar de São João, in Porto, Portugal recruited 112 men with a diagnosis of infertility at the first ART cycle. Participants completed the Inventory State-Trait Anxiety-Form Y (STAI-Y), the Beck Depression Inventory-II (BDI-II), the Dyadic Adjustment Scale (DAS), and the Fertility Problem Inventory (FPI) before the start of treatment. Anxiety status had a linear negative impact on slow progressive sperm motility ($p < 0.05$). This shows how psychopathological symptoms before an ART cycle can affect sperm motility.

However, this association seems to be present only in men undergoing ART treatments for the first time. Therefore, the need for mental health professionals to respond to the emotional difficulties of the male gender is increasingly emerging, through the development of appropriate psychological interventions, in order to minimize the impact of exposure to ART treatments.

12.3 Male Fragility

Similarly to women, men suffer both physically and psychologically due to fertility treatments. Although there is a vast body of evidence of women's emotional adaptation to infertility, there are no systematic reviews focused on men's psychological adaptation to infertility and related treatments.

From the beginning of one study, until September 2015, a bibliographic search was conducted on five databases using combinations of MeSH terms and keywords

[13]. Eligible studies had to present prospective quantitative designs and samples that included men who had not achieved pregnancy or parenthood at follow-up.

Results: Twelve studies from three continents were eligible among 2534 records identified in the search. The results revealed that psychological symptoms of maladjustment significantly increased in men 1 year after the first fertility assessment. No significant differences were found two or more years after the initial consultation. Evidence of anxiety, depression, active avoidance coping, catastrophizing, difficulties in communication with the partner and the use of avoidance or religious coping by the wife as risk factors for psychological maladjustment were found. Protective factors were related to the use of coping strategies that involved seeking information and attributing a positive meaning to infertility, support from others and one's spouse, and engagement in open communication about the infertility problem.

12.4 Do We Still Wonder What the Purpose of Psychosexual Counseling Is?

Adaptation, coping behavior, depression, infertility, marital relationship, men, women, protective and risk factors, psychology, fatigue, and systematic review are just some of the topics covered by the psychosexual counselor. This alone would favor the active involvement of men during the treatment process by health care providers, and the inclusion in counseling of training courses in coping skills and improving couple communication, as well as doctor–patient communication.

The prospective longitudinal study by Schmidt et al. [14] is proof of this: we are talking about a sample of 2250 people who had started fertility treatment with a 12-month follow-up. The data were based on self-administered questionnaires that measured communication with the partner and with other people. Coping strategies are active avoidance coping, active confrontation coping, passive avoidance coping, meaning-based coping, and stress from fertility problems. The study population included those participants (n = 816, men and women) who had not achieved a pregnancy through assisted reproduction or childbirth at follow-up.

Results: Among both men and women, difficulties in communication with the partner were predictive of high stress related to fertility problems (odds ratio for women, 3.47, 95% confidence interval = 2.09–5.76; odds ratio for men, 3.69, 95% confidence interval = 2.09–6.43). Active avoidance coping (e.g., avoiding being with pregnant women or children, focusing on work to distract the mind from things) was a significant predictor of high stress from fertility problems.

Among men, high use of active coping (e.g., venting feelings, asking advice from other people, seeking social support) predicted low stress related to fertility problems within the marital context (odds ratio 0.53, 95% confidence interval = 0.28–1.00).

Another study by Schmidt et al. [15] sought to investigate the marital benefit, which infertility could bring to the marriage by strengthening the partners who start a fertility treatment and communication and coping strategies as predictors of marital benefit 12 months later.

A total of 2250 people who had started fertility treatment and a 12-month follow-up were recruited. The data were based on self-administered questionnaires that measured marital benefit, communication, and coping strategies, without having achieved a childbirth after fertility treatment.

Results: 25.9% of women and 21.1% of men reported a high marital benefit. Among men, the average use of active confrontation-based coping (e.g., letting out feelings, asking advice from others) was a predictor of high marital benefit. Conversely, considering infertility as a secret experience, using active avoidance strategies (e.g., avoiding being with pregnant women or children, focusing on work to distract) produced (among men) significant predictors of low marital benefits.

12.5 The Female World

What about family stress among hospitalized women with ovarian hyperstimulation syndrome receiving treatment for infertility?

When hospitalization is necessary for infertile women with ovarian hyperstimulation syndrome, they must face transient stress between health and illness, and their families are traumatized by the pressure of hospitalization. Most of the literature on infertility treatment has focused on the physiopsychological reactions of infertile women, the impact on couple relationships, and the influence of social support on infertile couples.

In the study by Chang and Mu [16], ten married couples were recruited from a medical center in Taipei. All the couples were undergoing treatment for infertility. An open and in-depth interview technique encouraged the couples to reflect on their experience, bringing their feelings to a more conscious level. *Results*: This study explored the experiences of infertile women from the couples' perspective and the results identify the overall stress that the family must face. Five themes emerged: the stress of "carrying on the ancestral line," the couple's psychological reactions, the disruption of family life, the reorganization of family life, and external family support.

The results show that the experience of family stress involves impacts that range across the realms of individual, marital, family, and social interactions and that it is necessary to cope with these when the wife is hospitalized for moderate to severe ovarian hyperstimulation syndrome.

The cross-sectional study by Kim et al. [17] then identified the factors influencing the intention of continuous fertility treatments among women undergoing assisted reproduction technology (ART). A total of 197 women were recruited in fertility hospitals in Gyeonggi-do and Busan, South Korea. Data were collected using a self-report questionnaire that incorporated measures of uncertainty, Depression Anxiety Stress Scales; Fatigue Severity Scale; Women's Infertility

Coping Scale; spousal support; treatment environment; and intention of continuous fertility treatment.

Results: A full 70.6% of participants expressed the intention to undergo continuous fertility treatments. The analysis highlighted that this characteristic was more deep rooted in patients with a longer marriage. These results underline the importance of managing uncertainty, adopting proactive coping strategies, supportive treatment environments, and considering the duration of marriage in relation to women's intention to undergo continuous fertility treatment in the context of ART. The implications of these results extend to the development of psychosexual intervention programs aimed at providing crucial support to women undergoing ART and seeking to continue infertility treatment.

12.6 Research Questionnaires

Relationship satisfaction is the quantity and quality of a person's feelings about their intimate relationship [18]. As part of the relational satisfaction assessment, marriage quality was introduced as an overall marriage assessment in which factors such as various marriage characteristics, attitudes, behaviors, and communication patterns are used [19]. Some relational characteristics such as the level of satisfaction with the relationship, the type of attitudes toward the partner, and low levels of aggression and hostility can be used to investigate the quality of marriage. It has been shown that the quality of marriage is associated with health problems and well-being, feelings of happiness, economic factors, psychological complications, and general aspects of quality of life [20]. However, the assessment of marital quality among infertile patients involves psychological and mental health problems including depression, stress, anxiety, sexual dysfunctions, and poor marital satisfaction, well-being, and quality of life [21].

Numerous self-assessment tools have been introduced and used to assess marital quality such as the Marital Adjustment Test (MAT), the Kansas Marital Satisfaction Scale (KMSS), the Dyadic Adjustment Scale (DAS), the Couples Satisfaction Index (CSI), the Relationship Assessment Scale (RAS), Quality of Marriage Index (QMI) [22]. The QMI, developed by Norton [22] is a measure of marital satisfaction composed of six elements. This scale is useful for verifying the contribution of agreement in the relationship and the similarity of attitudes within couples. Moreover, the brevity of the tool compared to other tools can represent a considerable advantage so that it is possible to evaluate large populations in a short period of time.

12.7 Conclusions

The discontinuation of ART is an unresolved problem in fertility clinics. Many couples discontinue assisted reproduction technology (ART) pathways without achieving a live birth for reasons other than unfavorable prognosis or treatment cost. The suspension has been attributed to the burden of treatment. The causes of the burden can be broadly classified depending on whether they originate in the patient, the clinic, or the treatment. Interventions to alleviate these burdens include providing comprehensive educational material, screening to identify highly distressed patients, providing tailored coping tools, and improvements in the clinical environment and medical interventions. There are practical interventions to reduce the various causes of burden in ART, but further development and evaluation of the effectiveness of these interventions require a more precise definition of the theory.

Couples teach that there is not a single infertility from a psychosexual point of view, but an infertility for each type of couple. This should be referred to in counseling so that individuals do not feel passive or strangers during clinical treatments. The psychosexual therapist could also be useful to facilitate the couple's relationship with the medical team and among clinicians to propose a single communicative style and increase individual compliance.

In more structured centers, it is possible to schedule a team meeting to compare clinical and psychosexual information, as well as to agree on a communicative style with a positive connotation. Which is to say, to communicate even uncertain or failed diagnoses without pathologizing individuals and the couple. Giving them an assignment for a second couple project.

References

1. Macedo CM, Miura PO, Barrientos DMS, Lopes GA, Egry EY (2018) Coping strategies for domestic violence against pregnant adolescents: integrative review. Rev Bras Enferm 71(Suppl 1):693–699. https://doi.org/10.1590/0034-7167-2017-0682
2. Lazarus RS, Folkman S (1984) Stress, assessment and coping. Springer Publishing Company, New York
3. Folkman S (1997) Positive psychological states and management of severe stress. Soc Sci Med 45:1207–1221. https://doi.org/10.1016/s0277-9536(97)00040-3
4. Aflakseir A, Zarei M (2013) Association between coping strategies and infertility stress in a group of women with fertility problems in Shiraz, Iran. J Reprod Sterile 14:202–206
5. Peterson BD, Pirritano M, Christensen U, Schmidt L (2008) The impact of partner coping in couples suffering from infertility. Hum Reprod 23:1128–1137. https://doi.org/10.1093/humrep/den067
6. Kaya Z, Oskay U (2019) Stigma, despair, and coping experiences of Turkish women with infertility. J Reprod Child Psychol 38:485–496. https://doi.org/10.1080/02646838.2019.1650904
7. Zurlo MC, Cattaneo Della Volta MF, Vallone F (2020) Reexamining the role of coping strategies in associations between dimensions of infertility-related stress and state anxiety: implications for clinical interventions with infertile couples. Front Psychol 11:614887. https://doi.org/10.3389/fpsyg.2020.614887

8. Schick M, Roesner S, Germeyer A, Moessner M, Bauer S, Ditzen B, Wischmann T (2019) Positive adjustment coping intervention supported by smartphone (PACI) for couples undergoing fertility treatment: a randomized controlled study protocol. BMJ Open 9:e025288. https://doi.org/10.1136/bmjopen-2018-025288
9. Czamanski-Cohen J, Sarid O, Cwikel J, Levitas E, Har-Vardi I (2018) Are there preferred coping and communication strategies during in vitro fertilization and do cognitive behavioral interventions help? J Ment Health Train Educ Pract 14:20–30. https://doi.org/10.1108/JMHTEP-04-2018-0022
10. Valoriani V, Lotti F, Lari D, Miccinesi G, Vaiani S, Vanni C, Coccia ME, Maggi M, Noci I (2016) Differences in psychophysical Well-being and signs of depression in couples undergoing their first consultation for assisted reproduction technology (ART): an Italian pilot study. Eur J Obstet Gynecol Reprod Biol 197:179–185. https://doi.org/10.1016/j.ejogrb.2015.11.041. Epub 7. PMID: 26773309
11. Reis S, Xavier MR, Coelho R, Montenegro N (2016) Psychological impact of single and multiple courses of assisted reproductive treatments in couples: a comparative study. Eur J Obstet Gynecol Reprod Biol 171(1):61–66. https://doi.org/10.1016/j.ejogrb.2013.07.034. Epub 6. PMID: 23928476
12. Bártolo A, Reis S, Monteiro S, Leite R, Montenegro N (2013) Psychological adjustment of infertile men undergoing fertility treatments: an association with sperm parameters. Arch Psychiatr Nurs 30(5):521–526. https://doi.org/10.1016/j.apnu.2016.04.014. Epub 2016 Apr 30. PMID: 27654231
13. Martins MV, Basto-Pereira M, Pedro J, Peterson B, Almeida V, Schmidt L, Costa ME (2016) Male psychological adaptation to unsuccessful medically assisted reproduction treatments: a systematic review. Hum Reprod Update 22(4):466–478. https://doi.org/10.1093/humupd/dmw009. Epub 2016 Mar 23. PMID: 27008894
14. Schmidt L, Holstein BE, Christensen U, Boivin J (2005) Communication and coping as predictors of fertility problem stress: cohort study of 816 participants who did not achieve a delivery after 12 months of fertility treatment. Hum Reprod 20(11):3248–3256. https://doi.org/10.1093/humrep/dei193. Epub 2005 Jul 8. PMID: 16006458
15. Schmidt L, Holstein B, Christensen U, Boivin J (2005) Does infertility cause marital benefit? An epidemiological study of 2250 women and men in fertility treatment. Patient Educ Couns 59(3):244–251. https://doi.org/10.1016/j.pec.2005.07.015. Epub 2005 Nov 28. PMID: 16310331
16. Chang SN, Mu PF (2008) Infertile couples' experience of family stress while women are hospitalized for ovarian hyperstimulation syndrome during infertility treatment. J Clin Nurs 17(4):531–538. https://doi.org/10.1111/j.1365-2702.2006.01801.x. Epub 2007 Mar 1. PMID: 17331094
17. Kim M, Kim M, Ban M (2024) Factors influencing the intention for continual fertility treatments by the women undergoing assisted reproductive technology procedures: a cross-sectional study. J Korean Acad Nurs 54(1):59–72. Korean. PMID: 38480578. https://doi.org/10.4040/jkan.23095
18. Maroufizadeh S, Almasi-Hashiani A, Amini P, Sepidarkish M, Omani-Samani R (2019) The Quality of Marriage Index (QMI): a validation study in infertile patients. BMC Res Notes 12(1):507. https://doi.org/10.1186/s13104-019-4438-2. PMID: 31412948; PMCID: PMC6693237
19. Carr D, Freedman VA, Cornman JC, Schwarz N (2014) Happy marriage, happy life? Marital quality and subjective well-being in later life. J Marriage Fam 76(5):930–948
20. Liu H, Waite L (2014) Bad marriage, broken heart? Age and gender differences in the link between marital quality and cardiovascular risks among elders. J Health Soc Behav 55(4):403–423

21. Maroufizadeh S, Omani-Samani R, Bagheri-Lankarani N, Almasi-Hashiani A, Amini P (2018) Factors associated with poor well-being of infertile individuals: a cross-sectional study. Middle East Fert Soc J 23(4):468–470
22. Reynolds J, Houlston C, Coleman L (2014) Understanding relationship quality. OnePlus One, London

Chapter 13
Under the Sign of the Gemini

In recent decades, as a result of assisted reproduction technology (ART), the number of multiple pregnancies has increased in the United States [1]. Such pregnancies are associated with a higher rate of complications for both the mother and the child, as well as a range of social, psychological, and economic consequences.

Despite this, multiple pregnancies in general and twin pregnancies in particular are considered an adverse/unwanted effect of ART by reproductive medicine specialists. In 2015, almost half of all multiple pregnancies resulting from ART in the United States occurred in women under 35 years of age who had had two fresh or frozen blastocysts transferred [2].

The rates of multifetal pregnancies among young patients undergoing in vitro fertilization (IVF) remained high in 2016, with nearly 17% of women under 35 years of age having a live multifetal birth [3].

Subsequently, the frequency of twin births in the United States has consistently decreased since 2017, with a 3% decrease in twins from 2018 to 2019, and a 5% decrease compared to 33.9% in 2014 [4].

One of the main theories supporting this trend is the technological maturation of fertility treatments, which involves transferring a smaller number of embryos each cycle. This theory seems to be supported by the observed drop in twin rates resulting from in vitro fertilization treatment, from 12.8% for autologous retrieval in women under 35 years in 2017 to 7.3% for retrieval in the same age group in 2019 (SART success rate data).

Despite this decrease, the current rate of twins in the total population of the United States (born from in vitro fertilization treatment) is 31.5%. Furthermore, the annual rate of twins from ART in all age groups (4–9%) remains higher than the expected rate of twins from spontaneous conception (3.4%) [5].

Usually, in the United States, doctors and patients decide together how many embryos to transfer in in vitro fertilization cycles. All the more so as the American Society for Reproductive Medicine (ASRM) recommends, as an optimal outcome of ART, the implantation of a single fetus [6].

E. V. Longhi, *Framing Sexual Dysfunctions and Diseases during Fertility Treatment*, https://doi.org/10.1007/978-3-031-76726-5_13

Conversely, multifetal pregnancies include higher rates of preterm birth and perinatal complications including anemia, gestational diabetes, hypertensive disease of pregnancy, postpartum hemorrhage, and maternal mortality [7]. These complications are amplified by the mother's advanced age [8] all the more so as pregnancy occurs increasingly later in many countries, including the United States [9].

This is not to mention the maternal complications developed during pregnancy, including gestational hypertension, eclampsia and preeclampsia, gestational diabetes, placenta previa, placental abruption, placenta accreta, preterm birth (gestational age at birth, 28–36 weeks), dystocia, cesarean delivery, and postpartum hemorrhage (bleeding volume ≥500 mL after vaginal delivery or ≥1000 mL after cesarean delivery).

Last but not the least, the neonatal complications that can develop before or after birth until discharge, including fetal growth restriction (an estimated fetal weight during ultrasound screening that is below the tenth percentile of gestational age), low birth weight (<1500 g), macrosomia (birth weight >4000 g), malformations (congenital malformations, deformations, and chromosomal abnormalities), and stillbirth (death or loss of a child before or during delivery at 20 weeks of gestational age or later) [8].

13.1 Once upon a Time, There Was Sexuality

It should be added that in almost all of these couples, sexuality is a distant memory. The partner's premature or delayed ejaculation (or erectile dysfunction) often limited the frequency and quality of intimacy over time. Therefore, the choice to have twins can become the solution to His frustration and Her pacification. Especially when friends or siblings have already had children.

Sexuality at this point is "forgotten" just like "an unhappy sexual past." ART becomes the sole and exclusive purpose of the couple. Each individual in the couple feels "responsibilized" with respect to their sexual role, at least until postpartum.

Consequently, patients may not be aware of the risks associated with multiple pregnancies.

Twenty-nine percent of patients reported wanting a twin pregnancy before receiving appropriate information from clinicians, and 14% of couples continued with their desire for a twin pregnancy after an educational campaign [10].

The study by Griffin et al. [11] conducted in 2008–2009 found that greater understanding of the risks of a twin pregnancy led to the choice of a single pregnancy in 20.4% of patients who initially desired twin parenthood.

The relationship between greater knowledge and decreased desire for twins remains clear [12].

Multiple patient-level variables have been associated with the desire to have twins, including the desire to quickly complete family building, a decent family income, younger age, nulliparity, duration of infertility, and a previous fertility assessment [13].

Some studies have focused on specific complications such as preeclampsia, low birth weight, and postpartum depression in assessing the patient's knowledge of the risk of twins with infertility [14]. Other studies have asked a single question pertaining to awareness of the risks (i.e., "Do you consider that children born from a multiple pregnancy are at greater risk than single children?") [15].

It should be added that all these studies do not have a sexological history of the couple before the diagnosis of infertility, nor do we have postpartum sexological follow-ups.

13.2 What About the Rest of the World?

In 2005 the rate of single embryo transfer in Europe was about 20%, but in other countries much higher rates are recorded: 69% in Sweden (also in 2005) and 57% in Australia and New Zealand in 2006.

Data from the Cochrane database of 2014 showed that the live birth rate (LBR) following a single cycle of double embryo transfer was 45%, while the LBR following a single cycle of single embryo transfer was between 24% and 33%.

The LBR following repeated transfer of a single embryo would be between 31% and 44%.

The risk of having twins was about seven times higher after double embryo transfer [16].

In Sweden, in 2004, single embryo transfer (SET) accounted for 67% of all transfers, with an almost unchanged birth rate of 27% per transfer, while the IVF multiple birth rate had reduced to 5.6% [17].

The Turkish government has implemented new legislation starting from March 2010 in an attempt to promote the transfer of a single embryo. According to the new regulation, in the first and second cycle of treatment for patients under 35 years old, only one embryo transfer is allowed, in the third or subsequent cycles, a maximum of two embryos can be transferred and for patients over 35 years old, a maximum of two embryos can be transferred [18].

But there is more.

A study by Md Latar and Razali [19] found that among those who desired twin pregnancies, 46.7% of men and 44.8% of women justified their choice because of age. 11.1% of men and 15.5% of women interviewed, respectively, indicated the long duration of the attempt to conceive as a reason for preferring twin pregnancies. Other reasons given were the high cost of fertility treatment (2.2% vs. 5.1%), the desire to complete the family faster, concern about the inability or difficulty in getting pregnant again, or health factors.

13.3 The Risks of Art

Sexuality aside, some studies have shown that ART pregnancies present a higher risk of adverse outcomes. The risks demonstrated include an increase in rates of prematurity and low birth weight, as well as an increase in babies born "small" for gestational age [20].

It has been shown that pregnancies assisted by ART have an increased risk of preeclampsia, gestational diabetes, and hemorrhagic disorders [21].

Much of the increased risk associated with ART is due to multiple gestations [22]; however, the risks also increase in single pregnancies.

The reasons for the increase in adverse outcomes with ART are unknown. One hypothesis is that they derive from the ART procedure itself and are caused by drugs used to stimulate multiple ovulations, manipulations of gametes, in vitro cultures, transfer of multiple embryos, or other phenomena related to the treatment.

Another hypothesis is that the basic diagnoses related to the infertility of women undergoing ART directly contribute to adverse outcomes.

One historical study included 305,774 pregnancies with single and twin live births that occurred between July 1, 2004 and December 31, 2008 in Massachusetts.

The study population included live births of 3689 women with (following ART treatment) ART treatment and a single diagnosis of male factor, endometriosis, ovulation disorders, or tubal disease; 4098 women without ART treatment and with a single diagnosis of endometriosis, ovulation disorders, or reproductive inflammation; and 297,987 women without ART treatment nor with one of the above diagnoses. Overall, women treated with ART (34.5 ± 4.0 years) were significantly older compared to untreated women with ART with infertility-related diagnoses (26.3 ± 5.6 years) or fertile women (29.7 ± 5.8 years; $p < 0.0001$).

Birth certificate data of newborns and patient discharge data were obtained from the PELL data system. The PELL database was developed as a collaborative effort between the Department of Public Health of Massachusetts, the CDC, and the School of Public Health of Boston University and links the demographic data of birth certificates and fetal death, hospital discharges, and child health and development program data.

Pregnancy and newborn birth outcomes included maternal morbidity (hypertension in pregnancy and gestational diabetes), prenatal hospital use (emergency room visits, observational admissions, and hospital admissions), delivery complications (primary cesarean delivery), and birth outcomes (preterm birth, low birth weight, and small for gestational age). The control groups were births of fertile women.

From the birth certificates, we obtained uterine bleeding, placental abruption, excessive bleeding during labor, placenta previa, breech presentation and malpresentation, cephalopelvic disproportion, and mode of delivery. Pregnancy hypertension and gestational diabetes were identified from the birth certificate or from the hospital discharge record (ICD-9 codes 642 for pregnancy-related hypertension; 648.8 for gestational diabetes).

Results: All types of infertility treated with and without ART, except those with reproductive inflammation, had a higher rate of cesarean section compared to births of fertile women. Gestational diabetes, hospital admissions, preterm births, and low birth weight were all increased in both the ART-treated and non-ART-treated groups for this study group [22].

13.4 Conclusions

More than 10 years have passed since the last study published on the desire for twins in patients with infertility in the United States. The long period of COVID, and the consequent inability to access specialized fertility centers, has caused a "void" in couple's sexuality in general and in plans for the future.

It is clear that many patients still desire twins today, despite the continuous expansion of insurance mandates, the advances in the effectiveness of ART, and knowledge of the inherent risks of multiple pregnancies. It is also clear that efforts focused exclusively on reducing the desire for twins are an inefficient strategy to effectively reduce twin pregnancies motivated more by the patient's anxiety about family growth than by a clear assessment of the physical, psychological, and relational risks of the patient and the couple.

References

1. Mendoza R, Jáuregui T, Diaz-Nuñez M, de la Sota M, Hidalgo A, Ferrando M, Martínez-Indart L, Expósito A, Matorras R (2018) Infertile couples prefer twins: analysis of their reasons and clinical characteristics related to this preference. J Reprod Infertil 19(3):167–173
2. Kissin DM, Kulkarni AD, Mneimneh A, Warner L, Boulet SL, Crawford S et al (2015) Embryo transfer practices and multiple births resulting from assisted reproduction technologies: a prevention opportunity. Fertil Sterile 103:954–961. https://doi.org/10.1016/j.fertnstert.2014.12.127
3. Society for Assisted Reproductive Technology. National summary report. Available at: https://www.sartcorsonline.com/rptCSR_PublicMultYear. aspx?reportingYear1/42019. Accessed on 18 Nov 2021
4. Martin JA, Hamilton BE, Osterman MJK, Driscoll AK (2021) Births: final data 2019. National vital statistics reports; vol 70 no. 2. National Center for Health Statistics, Hyattsville
5. Sunderam S, Kissin DM, Zhang Y, Folger SG, Boulet SL, Warner L, Callaghan WM, Barfield WD (2019) Surveillance of assisted reproductive technologies—United States, 2016. MMWR Surveill Summ 68(4):1–23. https://doi.org/10.15585/mmwr.ss6804a1
6. (2021) Practice Committee of the American Society for Reproductive Medicine and Practice Committee of the Society for Assisted Reproductive Technologies Guidelines on the limits to the number of embryos to transfer: committee opinion. Fertil Sterile 116(3):651–654. https://doi.org/10.1016/j.fertnstert.2021.06.050
7. Santana DS, Cecatti JG, Surita FG, Silveira C, Costa ML, Souza JP, Mazhar SB, Jayaratne K, Qureshi Z, Sousa MH, Vogel JP, WHO Multicountry Survey on Maternal and Newborn Health Research Network (2016) Twin pregnancy and severe maternal illness outcomes: the World

Health Organization's multinational survey on maternal and newborn health. Obstet Gynecol 127(4):631–641. https://doi.org/10.1097/AOG.0000000000001338
8. Wang Y, Shi H, Chen L, Zheng D, Long X, Zhang Y, Wang H, Shi Y, Zhao Y, Wei Y, Qiao J (2021) Absolute risk of adverse obstetric outcomes among twin pregnancies after in vitro fertilization by maternal age. JAMA Netw Open 4(9):e2123634. https://doi.org/10.1001/jamanetworkopen.2021.23634
9. Adashi EY, Gutman R (2021) Delayed pregnancy as a growing, previously unrecognized, factor to the excess of plural births nationally. Obstet Gynecol 132(4):999–1006. https://doi.org/10.1097/AOG.0000000000002853
10. Ryan GL, Sparks AE, Sipe CS, Syrop CH, Dokras A, Van Voorhis BJ (2007) A mandatory single blastocyst transfer policy with an educational campaign in a United States in vitro fertilization program reduces multiple gestation rates without sacrificing pregnancy rates. Fertil Steril 88(2):354–360. https://doi.org/10.1016/j.fertnstert.2007.03.001
11. Griffin D, Brown L, Feinn R, Jacob MC, Scranton V, Egan J, Nulsen J (2012) Impact of an educational intervention and insurance coverage on patient preferences for multiple embryo transfers. Reprod Biomed Online 25(2):204–208. https://doi.org/10.1016/j.rbmo.2012.04.006
12. Murray S, Shetty A, Rattray A, Taylor V, Bhattacharya S (2004) A randomized comparison of alternative methods of information provision on the acceptability of elective single embryo transfer. Hum Reprod 19(4):911–916. https://doi.org/10.1093/humrep/deh176
13. Ryan GL, Zhang SH, Dokras A, Syrop CH, Van Voorhis BJ (2004) The desire of infertile patients for multiple births. Fertil Steril 81:500–504. https://doi.org/10.1016/j.fertnstert.2003.05.035
14. Newton CR, McBride J, Feyles V, Tekpetey F, Power S (2007) Factors influencing patient attitudes towards single and multiple embryo transfers. Fertil Steril 87(2):269–278. https://doi.org/10.1016/j.fertnstert.2006.06.043
15. Child TJ, Henderson AM, Tan SL (2004) The desire for multiple pregnancies in patients with male and female infertility. Hum Reprod 19:558–561. https://doi.org/10.1093/humrep/deh097
16. American Society for Reproductive Medicine (2012) Elective single embryo transfer. Fertil Steril 97:835–842
17. Bergh C, Kjellberg AT, Karlstrom PO (2005) Fertilization of a single in vitro embryo. Birth rate maintained despite the drastically reduced frequency of multiple births. Lakartidningen 102:3444–3447
18. Urman B, Yakin K (2010) New Turkish legislation on techniques and assisted reproduction centers: a step in the right direction? Reprod Biomed Online 21(6):729–731
19. Md Latar IL, Razali N (2014) The desire for multiple pregnancy among patients with infertility and their partners. Int J Reprod Med 2014:301452. https://doi.org/10.1155/2014/301452
20. Luke B, Stern JE, Kotelchuck M, Hornstein MD, Declercq E, Cohen B et al (2014) Birth outcomes through infertility treatment: analysis of the Massachusetts Outcomes Study of Assisted Reproductive Technologies (MOSART). Fertil Steril 102:e17
21. Declercq E, Belanoff C, Diop H, Gopal D, Hornstein MD, Kotelchuck M et al (2014) Identifying women with indicators of subfertility in a state-level population database: operationalizing the missing link in ART research. Fertil Steril 101:463–471
22. Grigorescu V, Zhang Y, Kissin DM, Sauber-Schatz E, Sunderam M, Kirby RS et al (2014) Maternal characteristics and pregnancy outcomes after assisted reproduction technology by infertility diagnosis: ovulatory dysfunction versus tubal obstruction. Fertil Steril 101:1019–1025

Chapter 14
In Vitro Fertilization: Sexuality and Pregnancy

After the long medical preparatory process and the stress of waiting for the results of fertilization procedures, every pregnant woman undergoes changes in endocrine function, anatomical changes, and psychosomatic symptoms that mark each trimester of pregnancy, limiting her sexual response [1]. The increase in prolactin and oxytocin levels during pregnancy indirectly influence genital arousal and subjective sexual arousal, while perceived anxiety and stress can negatively affect desire, passion, and quality of life. However, higher levels of estrogen and progesterone in the second trimester increase blood flow to the genitals and can lead to an increase [2] in sexual desire. The process of building motherhood involves a lot of anxiety and primal fears, such as doubts about labor, the ability to produce a healthy child, and new relationships with the arrival of a new family member. In addition to this process, there are still adjustments to the new body, physical discomfort, and fatigue, which, combined with cultural factors, can affect the couple's sexual life [3].

According to a Brazilian review [4], the prevalence of sexual dysfunction during pregnancy ranged from 38.9% to 73.3%, depending on the trimester of pregnancy evaluated and on associated diseases [5]. As pregnancy progressed, sexual practice progressively lost frequency and quality of intercourse: particularly in desire, arousal, lubrication, orgasm, satisfaction, and dyspareunia [6].

Female sexual dysfunctions are often associated with individual variables: some studies highlight maternal age, education, pregnancy planning, body image, satisfaction with the couple's relationship, depression, and anxiety [7]. However, there is no established evidence of the real influence of most of these factors on sexual function.

On the other hand, it is clear that sexuality before pregnancy plays an important role in maintaining sexuality during pregnancy [8].

In this context, assessing a couple's sexual function from the beginning of pregnancy could be useful in maintaining healthy sexual activity, reducing and alleviating any anxiety. Moreover, it is essential to know the main changes resulting from

E. V. Longhi, *Framing Sexual Dysfunctions and Diseases during Fertility Treatment*, https://doi.org/10.1007/978-3-031-76726-5_14

pregnancy in order to apply measures aimed at minimizing the impact of sexual dysfunctions on the couple's relationship.

The search for further epidemiological data evaluating the prevalence of sexual dysfunctions before and during pregnancy, as well as the factors associated with them, is important to measure the extent of this problem.

14.1 Research Questionnaires

Barclay et al. [9], for example, developed the Pregnancy and Sexuality Questionnaire (PSQ), a validated tool for studying sexual relations between partners during pregnancy.

Rudge et al. [8] have, on the other hand, designed and validated a Pregnancy Sexual Response Inventory (PSRI) to assess changes in sexuality during pregnancy, in short form, useful for both low- and high-risk pregnancies. The research process was conducted at the Department of Obstetrics and Gynecology of the Faculty of Medicine of Botucatu, State University of Sao Paulo (UNESP), Brazil. Approval for the study was given by the local Institutional Research Board (IRB) and a written informed consent statement was obtained from all participants before the interview. Women with a single pregnancy between 10 and 35 weeks of gestation were contacted, distributed approximately evenly in the three trimesters of pregnancy. The final PSRI was divided into ten domains, eight of which related to the woman's feelings and two to her perception of her partner.

The ten domains of female feelings included:

(a) Frequency: a three-item scale that assessed the frequency of sexual intercourse relative to pregnancy;
(b) Desire: a three-item scale that assessed the frequency of desire before and during pregnancy and the frequency of participation in sexual activity;
(c) Arousal: a three-item scale that assessed the quality of sexual activity before and during pregnancy;
(d) Orgasm: a three-item scale that assessed the frequency of orgasm before and during pregnancy;
(e) Pleasure: a three-item scale that assessed the enjoyment of sexual life before and during pregnancy;
(f) Dyspareunia: a two-item scale that assessed the pain during sexual intercourse before and during pregnancy;
(g) Initiation of intercourse: a three-item scale that assessed the start of participation in sexual activity before and during pregnancy;
(h) Female sexual difficulties: a two-item scale that assessed any female sexual difficulties before and during pregnancy. The woman's perception of her partner's sexuality included;
(i) Male sexual pleasure: a three-item scale that assessed the female view of male pleasure before and during pregnancy;

(j) Male sexual difficulties: a two-item scale that assessed the female view of male sexual difficulties before and during pregnancy.

In summary, the PSRI appears to be a clinical tool composed of 38 items (12 demographic characteristics and 26 sexual behaviors/activities) that provides a brief semi-structured interview to assess the impact of pregnancy on sexuality. Clinicians and sexologists can benefit from it, always bearing in mind that each pregnancy and each couple describes a story of feelings, stress, and difficulties that should not be underestimated.

14.2 The Study with the PSRI

An application of the PSRI is found in a study in which 262 pregnant women aged between 18 and 43 years were recruited, with an average age of 27.6 years and an average gestational age of 25.5 weeks. Of these, 7.2% were in the first trimester, 48.1% in the second, and 44.7% in the third [10].

The majority were married women (formally or informally, 82.8%), graduates (61.1%), and employees (47.7%). As for religion, 43.1% were Protestant and 40.8% Catholic. In relation to the number of children, 53.4% were first-time mothers and only 18.7% had two or more children. A total of 74.0% reported not using condoms, 96.2% did not consume alcohol, 99.2% did not smoke, and none reported using illicit drugs.

Results: A decrease in sexual activity was reported by 64.9% of women during pregnancy, while only 7.6% reported an increase in frequency. Sexual satisfaction during pregnancy decreased in 41.6% of women. A total of 92% reported being sexually satisfied before pregnancy and 50.8% during pregnancy. In terms of sexual desire, most participants reported that it depended on the occasion or predisposition. Regarding arousal, 80.9% of the sample rated it as excellent/good before pregnancy, dropping to 30.5% during pregnancy, while 0.4% rated it as bad/terrible before pregnancy, increasing to 23.3% during pregnancy.

When asked if they had orgasms during sexual intercourse, 90.1% responded that they always/usually did before pregnancy, while only 54.6% always/usually had orgasms during pregnancy. Dyspareunia was reported by 11.1% of women before pregnancy and by 45.8% during pregnancy. In the sample, 90.1% of pregnant women reported that the initiation of sexual intercourse was spontaneous before pregnancy, reducing to 68.7% after pregnancy. With pregnancy, the frequency of sexual difficulties/dysfunctions also increases, from 5.7% to 58.7%.

Finally, two areas of the questionnaire concerned the perception that pregnant women had about their partner's sexuality. Before pregnancy, 87.4% of the sample gave scores from 8 to 10 to partners in satisfaction and sexual response, while during pregnancy only 33.2% gave the same scores. Before pregnancy, only 1.1% reported that the partner had some sexual difficulty, but this rate increased to 10.3% during pregnancy.

Finally, regarding the association of sexual dissatisfaction with independent variables (maternal age, gestational age, couple status, education, religion, professional condition, number of children, use of condoms, pregnancy planning, smoking, and use of alcohol or drugs), the only variable associated with sexual dissatisfaction was education. A higher level of education reduced the possibility of being sexually dissatisfied by 50% and reported relationship problems in the couple.

14.3 Psyche and Sex

A recent study estimated that the prevalence of sexual dysfunction during pregnancy was 81% based on a limit score of the Female Sexual Function Index (FSFI) [11] of 26.55. Another study on sexual function during pregnancy in Poland found that pregnant women were more sexually active in the second trimester of pregnancy and that sexual function significantly decreased in the third trimester [12]. Sexual experiences during pregnancy can promote commitment, love, trust, and intimacy between a couple. Also, engagement in safe sexual activities during pregnancy is a fundamental element for couples during the transition from being partners to being parents. Unfortunately, many studies [13] show that pregnancy is linked to a decrease in sexual desire, a reduced frequency of sexual activity, less sexual satisfaction, fewer intimate relationships, and a higher incidence of problematic vaginismus.

Where does in vitro fertilization (IVF) fit into all of this? (It involves ovulation induction, egg retrieval, and embryo implantation.) [14]. It is no coincidence that an increasing number of infertile couples are currently [15] requesting in vitro fertilization treatment.

Drugs to counter infertility used during assisted reproduction technologies, scheduled sexual intercourse, the higher risk of miscarriage in the first trimester, and psychological factors can have a strong impact on the sexual function of these patients. This is because women with fertility problems usually prioritize infertility treatment and rarely seek help [16] for sexual problems.

In this regard, a study by Karakas and Aslan [16] recruited 70 women with primary infertility, of whom 35 were in the experimental group and 35 in the control group. The Female Sexual Function Scale and the Golombok-Rust Sexual Satisfaction Scale were administered during the initial and final evaluation. The experimental group was provided with two sessions of sexual counseling.

After counseling, there was a statistically significant improvement in the average scores for the Female Sexual Function Scale and in the total scores for the Golombok-Rust Sexual Satisfaction Scale. Women who had experienced infertility for 6 years and more had lesser improvements in sexual dysfunction and sexual dissatisfaction. Sexual counseling ultimately proved effective in improving sexual function and sexual satisfaction in women with 1 or 2 years of infertility.

14.4 The Value of Sexual Counseling [17]

Infertility is a multifactorial problem and many couples do not have sufficient knowledge and skills to adequately manage this experience. In recent years, considerable attention has been paid to the role of the psychological aspects of infertility and medical knowledge suggests a link between infertility and psychological factors [18]. The analysis of correlations found significant positive correlations between sexual dissatisfaction and sexual- and infertility-related concerns in couples [19].

In Iranian infertile couples, the most common psychological and emotional problems are dissatisfaction, frustration, anxiety, and fear [20]. Stress, depression, low self-esteem, marital dissatisfaction, sexual dissatisfaction, impairment of marital quality, a decrease in intimacy, fear of ending a marital relationship, impotence, and manifestations of clinical depression have been reported as psychological consequences of infertility [21]. The decrease in sexual satisfaction, for any reason (psychological, relational, social, etc.), has many negative consequences. During infertility treatment, 50–60% of couples reported a marked decrease in sexual satisfaction [15]. Sexual counseling can therefore influence the quality of sexual relations, leading to greater satisfaction in intimacy between couples and can increase their pleasure and relational bonding.

Psychological treatments, along with infertility treatment programs, increase mental health, make infertile people more resistant to stress, increase the effectiveness of infertility treatments and pursue infertile people for follow-up treatments. Mindfulness-based cognitive therapy is a recent development of cognitive therapy that is a short-term structured intervention based on the model of reduction of the cognitive therapy model [22].

A Master's in Obstetric Counseling with Code 6425 has been approved by the Ethics Committee of Shahid Sadoughi University of Medical Sciences, Yazd, Iran. In this study, ethical issues such as informed consent, privacy, confidentiality, and anonymity were considered. (In Iran, the husband also signs the informed consent.) [18].

A study with the following inclusion criteria was set up: diagnosis of infertility for at least 1 year; being the only wife of a man; being in their first marriage; living in Yazd, Iran; having reading and writing skills; being aged between 22 and 49 years; not participating in provisional sessions or other psychological interventions simultaneously during the study (if not those offered by the program itself). Again, the exclusion criteria included the history of mental illness as reported by the patient, taking psychiatric drugs, having chronic diseases, addiction, and the husband's diabetes.

All participants, 44 women, completed a sociodemographic questionnaire [22] and a sexual satisfaction questionnaire [23]. The questionnaire consisted of 25 questions, with 5-point scale responses and a 1–5 Likert scale. The study aimed to determine and compare the average score of sexual satisfaction in women suffering from infertility before the intervention (baseline), after the intervention (8th week), and follow-up (12th week).

The average sexual satisfaction score of women suffering from infertility in the intervention group was 62.9 ± 7.32, 71.6 ± 5.95, and 70.9 ± 6.26, before the intervention (baseline), after the intervention (8th week), and follow-up (12th week), respectively.

The average sexual satisfaction score of women suffering from infertility in the control group was 63.3 ± 6.82, 64.2 ± 7.93, and 62.25 ± 7.99 at baseline, 8th week after and after follow-up (12th week, respectively).

The results showed that in the intervention group, the average score of sexual satisfaction improved after the psychological intervention (8th week) ($p < 0.001$) and in the follow-up period ($p < 0.001$) (12th week).

14.5 Conclusions

Many studies recommend psychological counseling on sexual health for women suffering from infertility. One study showed that mindfulness-based cognitive therapy reduces anxiety, stress, and depression; other research referring to the BASNEF model highlights an increase in sexual relationship satisfaction in women with infertility [24]. Another study suggested sexual counseling based on the BETTER model in women with primary infertility and sexual dysfunction [16]. Evaluating these studies, it can be stated that any psychological intervention improves the sexual response of women suffering from infertility. In addition to improving perception of their own bodies in physical, mental, social, and environmental terms [25].

In the Iranian study, there were eight psychological sessions for each recruited woman. It is no coincidence that most of the participants in the study requested to continue the psychological meeting program.

References

1. Saotome TT, Yonezawa K, Suganuma N (2018) Sexual dysfunction and satisfaction in Japanese couples during pregnancy and postpartum. Sex Med 6:348–355
2. Schock H, Zeleniuch-Jacquotte A, Lundin E, Grankvist K, Lakso HÅ, Idahl A, Lehtinen M, Surcel HM, Fortner RT (2016) Hormone concentrations throughout uncomplicated pregnancies: a longitudinal study. BMC Pregnancy Childbirth 16:146
3. Asselmann E, Hoyer J, Wittchen HU, Martini J (2016) Sexual problems during pregnancy and after childbirth among women with and without anxiety and depressive disorders before pregnancy: a prospective longitudinal study. J Sex Med 13(01):95–104. https://doi.org/10.1016/j.jsxm.2015.12.005
4. Wolpe RE, Zomkowski K, Silva FP, Queiroz APA, Sperandio FF (2017) Prevalence of female sexual dysfunction in Brazil: a systematic review. Eur J Obstet Gynecol Reprod Biol 211:26–32. https://doi.org/10.1016/j.ejogrb.2017.01.018
5. Prado DS, Lima RV, de Lima LM (2013) [Impact of pregnancy on female sexual function]. Rev Bras Ginecol Obstet 35(05):205–209. https://doi.org/10.1590/S0100-72032013000500003

6. Pauls RN, Occhino JA, Dryfhout VL (2008) Effects of pregnancy on female sexual function and body image: a prospective study. J Sex Med 5(08):1915–1922. https://doi.org/10.1111/j.1743-6109.2008.00884.x
7. Yıldız H (2015) The relationship between pre-pregnancy sexuality and sexual function during pregnancy and the postpartum period: a prospective study. J Sex Marital Ther 41(01):49–59. https://doi.org/10.1080/0092623X.2013.811452
8. Rudge CVC, Calderon IMP, Dias A et al (2009) CCBY. Design and validity of a questionnaire to assess sexuality in pregnant women. Reprod Health 6:12. https://doi.org/10.1186/1742-4755-6-12
9. Barclay L, Bond M, Clark M (1992) Development of a tool to study the sexual relationship of partners during pregnancy. Aust J Adv Nurs 10:14–21
10. Guendler JA, Katz L, Flamini MEDM, Lemos A, Amorim MM (2019) Prevalence of sexual dysfunctions and their associated factors in pregnant women in an outpatient prenatal care clinic. Rev Bras Ginecol Obstet 41(9):555–563. https://doi.org/10.1055/s-0039-1695021. English
11. Daud S, Zahid AZM, Mohamad M, Abdullah B, Mohamad NAN (2019) Prevalence of sexual dysfunction in pregnancy. Arch Gynecol Obstet 300(5):1279–1285. https://doi.org/10.1007/s00404-019-05273-y
12. Sagiv-Reiss DM, Bimbaum GE, Safir MP (2012) Changes in sexual experiences and relationship quality during pregnancy. Arch Sex Behav 41:1241–1251
13. Khalesi ZB, Bokaie M, Attari SM (2018) Effect of pregnancy on sexual function of couples. Afr Health Sci 18:227–234
14. Hilbert SM (2019) Complications of assisted reproduction technology. Emerg Med Clin North Am 37:239–249
15. Sunderam S, Kissin DM, Crawford SB, Folger SG, Boulet SL, Warner L, Barfield WD (2018) Assisted Reproductive Technology Surveillance—United States, 2015. MMWR Surveill Summ 67:1–28
16. Karakas K, Aslan E (2019) Sexual counseling in women with primary infertility and sexual dysfunction: use of the BETTER model. J Sex Marital Ther 45(1):21–30. https://doi.org/10.1080/0092623X.2018.1474407. Epub 2019 Apr 3
17. Hosseini Nejad S, Bokaie M, Mojtaba Yassini Ardekani S (2023) Effectiveness of sexual health counseling based on mindfulness approach on sexual satisfaction in women suffering from infertility: an RCT. Int J Reprod Biomed 21(2):147–158. https://doi.org/10.18502/ijrm.v21i2.12805
18. Abedi Shargh N, Bakhshani NM, Mohebbi MD, Mahmudian K, Ahovan M, Mokhtari M et al (2016) The effectiveness of group cognitive therapy based on mindfulness on marital satisfaction and general health in women with infertility. Glob J Health Sci 8:230–235
19. Luk BHK, Loke AY (2019) Sexual satisfaction, intimacy and relationship of couples undergoing treatment for infertility. J Reprod Infant Psychol 37:108–122
20. Marvi N, Golmakani N, Heidarian Miri H, Esmaily H (2019) The effect of sex education based on the sexual health model on the sexual function of women with infertility. Iran J Nurs Midwifery Res 24:444–450
21. Ozturk S, Sut HK, Kucuk L (2019) Examination of sexual functions and depressive symptoms among infertile and fertile women. Pak J Med Sci 35:1355–1360
22. Sadeghi M, Farajkhoda T, Khanabadi M, Eftekhar M (2022) PERMA model versus integrative-behavioral couple therapy for fertility problems: a randomized clinical trial protocol. Int J Reprod BioMed 19:1105–1116
23. Larson JH, Anderson SM, Holman TB, Niemann BK (1998) A longitudinal study on the effects of premarital communication, relational stability, and self-esteem on sexual satisfaction in the first year of marriage. J Marital Sex there 24:193–206
24. Shahbazi A, Behboodi Moghadam Z, Maasoumi R, Saffari M, Mohammadi S, Montazeri A (2020) Effect of a health education program based on the BASNEF model of overall satisfac-

tion for sexual health and satisfaction for the quality of the sexual relationship among women with infertility. Int J Women's Health 12:975–982

25. Farajkhoda T, Ashrafi F, Bokaie M, Zareei Mahmoodabadi H (2021) Online versus face-to-face training program for improving sexual intimacy, counseling with cognitive-behavioral approach on sexual intimacy in pregnant women. J Marital Sex Ther 47:446–459

Chapter 15
Him, Her and the Families of Origin… Internet, Video, Forum, Facebook, Twitter

Chronic diseases for many patients, couples, and families of origin become a relational, social, and therapeutic aggregator. A kind of new emotional contract where the diagnosis and therapies are experienced by each individual (of the couple or of the families of origin) to eradicate or contain the pathology. However, a diagnosis of infertility causes isolation, inadequacy, embarrassment, shame and blame. People refrain from sharing their anxiety with friends, colleagues, acquaintances, and especially with parents. They fear criticism, judgment, disappointment, and misunderstanding.

Mothers often sense that the couple is not going through an easy time, but are more inclined to consider a crisis between the two, or a work problem, rather than their having difficulty conceiving. If the absences from Sunday lunches or the lack of their children's availability is justified by "we are having medical checks," then the parents may seem unemotional:

"You're too old now …you should have thought about it earlier…," "I gave birth to you healthy, don't come and tell me that your spermogram is my or your father's fault…" "Maybe it's your wife who doesn't have the right characteristics…you are athletic, healthy…it's nothing to do with you…" "Your sister gave birth after the first year of marriage, why do you have to give us such problems?"

Or too superstitious and apprehensive:

"Don't tell anyone, most people wouldn't understand…" "Don't tell mom, she's too sensitive…" "I'll take you to the appointments, you need me, your father is not suitable and your husband is always working…" "talk to that friend of yours who had twins and went to the Clinic…She knows more than us, …we have never known such a thing."

Many women feel responsible for their infertility, often devaluing the value of their femininity. "Maybe with another woman, my husband would become a father …" or they blame their sporting passions because if they had not been so keen on training, they would be more ready to have children. Hence, the obsession with

E. V. Longhi, *Framing Sexual Dysfunctions and Diseases during Fertility Treatment*, https://doi.org/10.1007/978-3-031-76726-5_15

online research to understand causes, solutions, percentages of failure–success in treatments for infertility.

Clinical experience shows that women undergoing fertility treatments link their anxiety to the success of the numerous medical procedures they were subjected to, while patients who had only struggled to conceive without medical intervention reported being very focused on the different phases of their menstrual cycle, the outcome of the same, delays, calculation of fertile days. This excessive mental energy dedicated to everything related to infertility often leads to a decrease in commitment to activities that were previously enjoyed and an increase in social withdrawal. Infertile partners often become victims of themselves, prone to self-blame, frustration, disappointment, and fear of causing a crisis in the couple [1]. Not surprisingly.

Infertility for many couples marks a process of general verification of couple expectations. Presenting oneself at an Infertility Center for many partners represents a first attempt to gather information and then to make a decision on what to do. The conflict occurs precisely over the level of priorities of individual needs and wants often not shared. Symmetrical struggles are observed between which of the two partners has suffered more, has always mediated, and has sacrificed in silence. Or conversely, couples become more complicated, united, emotionally involved, protective like "two chestnuts inside their casing." Couples have explained that relationships with friends and family often become tense in the context of infertility, partly because of the barrage of unnecessary comments and questions received from well-meaning loved ones. Even in the presence of a network of friends, phrases such as "there'll be a happy ending, you'll see" and "don't worry, everyone does it" are experienced as useless and circumstantial phrases, without a real purpose of complicity.

Martins et al. [2] studied a sample of 613 Portuguese patients interviewed online for a period of 3 months and in a fertility clinic for another 11 months. The research sought to verify how much the support of friends and family (in the therapeutic journey of infertility) was perceived by the men and women of the sample. The couples lived together for an average of 6 ± 3.5 years and had tried for a pregnancy for 3.8 ± 2.6 years. Almost half of the couples had undergone infertility treatments (41.3%). It was found that infertility stress was associated with low family support for women ($\beta = -0.27$, $p = 0.003$) and low partner support for both men and women. The support perceived by friends of both women and men was not significantly correlated with stress related to male or female infertility. Male infertility stress was also associated with poor family support. The variance of infertility stress was greater in women than in men.

The research by Frick-Bruder [3] concluded that only if the couple can accept that both the desire to have a child and their own infertility are deeply rooted in their relationship, will they be prepared to undergo and tolerate the stress and tensions related to fertility treatment without allowing it to completely govern their lives. If the doctor and the couple refuse to admit that there are limits and fail to recognize their own feelings of inadequacy and powerlessness (as well as the anger and sadness that inevitably follow), the couple will have no chance to free themselves and face the outcomes of medical therapy.

Furthermore, the study by Walen and Lachman [4] examined a sample of 2348 adults (55% male) aged between 25 and 75 years ($M = 46.3$), with experience of previous infertility, married, or cohabiting. Positive and negative social exchanges were more strongly linked to psychological well-being than to health. For both sexes, support, partner tension, and support from the family of origin were predictive of well-being measures. However, the most conditioning family strain appeared to be that on the female side compared to the parents of male patients.

The scientific literature agrees in showing that men and women are emotionally affected by the state of infertility in correlation to the perceived support of the partner. In women, in particular, although the association between family support and infertility stress was significant, the effect of partner support appears to be particularly high. This result is consistent with existing studies on the positive influence of partner support on fertility stress in women. The result is not surprising given that the marital relationship is one of the main sources of support in times of infertility stress in women and depression in men.

The study by Lund et al. [5] examined 695 participants (355 women and 340 men) who had failed medical treatment on severe depressive aspects. The questionnaire Mental Health Inventory 5 of the Short-Form 36 was administered, which included items on depressive symptoms and on support from friends and relatives in dealing with infertility.

Results: 15% of women and 6% of men undergoing unsuccessful treatment reported severe depressive symptoms. Among men, low emotional support and appreciation from the partner, as well as her high demands seemed to be the major causes of severe depression. Among women and men, low appreciation from the family of origin, conflicts and excessive demands from parents, friends, and acquaintances were determinants in bringing out severe depressive symptoms. Moreover, more women than men report severe depressive symptoms after 1 year of unsuccessful treatment. It is important to be aware of the possible negative impact of relational tension between patients with fertility who have received unsuccessful treatment [6].

15.1 Infertility and the Internet

We must also ask ourselves: How much do these couples trust the information reported by specialists, nurses, and staff of infertility clinics?

Even if the clinical information was exhaustive, scientific research has shown that women of different age groups interact more than men with online health information sources in countries such as the United States of America (USA), Germany, France, and European Union member states [7]. European Internet users show a greater propensity toward a more intensive use of eHealth if they resided in other European Union countries or outside the European Union and if they were born outside the European Union. Similarly, the residence of European Internet users in densely populated areas (cities or large inhabited centers) predicts greater use of eHealth. In this context, a fairer promotion of the use of eHealth in Europe should also consider the territorial dimension, with particular attention to the connection of national health systems and to a greater presence and use of the Internet in less densely populated areas. The importance that these sources have for infertile women or in the early years of motherhood has been the focus of more detailed research on women's engagement. Many women in developed countries describe being constantly online to obtain information and peer support on pregnancy and the care of infants and small children [8].

Studies suggest that most couples who turn to fertility clinics seek further information. They actively scour the media for relevant articles, read books and magazines, and search the Internet for tips and support [9]. One of the few studies [8] aimed at examining the information needs of infertile couples and the use they make of the information obtained in this way during the subsequent decision-making process, suggests that information seeking is the second step that couples take after recognizing that they have a problem. In a study on Canadian patients with infertility [10], it was found that 56% of current internet users had obtained information on fertility problems from the Internet, regardless of their socioeconomic or medical status. Of these, 30% found it useful in the decision-making process. Another Canadian study [11] reported greater use of the Internet among women, higher socioeconomic, and higher incomes groups. Himmel et al. [12] found that 66% of respondents visiting an "expert forum on the Internet on involuntary childlessness" expected general information on causes, conception, or an evaluation of drugs and 41% expected to discuss their actual treatment.

At the heart of every couple, however, there is the desire to have a child naturally and, if that should not be possible, they conceptualize their efforts in gathering information and changing their lifestyle as a contribution to their success or failure.

In fact, the search for useful information also reveals to them the potential benefits of support groups and alternative therapies such as reflexology and acupuncture. Moreover, couples seem to believe that this is an effective strategy. Those who became pregnant often felt that their actions could have helped them, relaxing the mind and body enough to be able to conceive. Those who were unable to help themselves, for example by losing weight, felt they had "sabotaged" their chances of getting pregnant. In the context of a longitudinal study, infertile couples blamed themselves for not doing what they could to maximize their chances of success [13]. Couples feel positive and empowered due to their efforts to pursue practices and lifestyles conducive to pregnancy. Even those who had tube damage or sperm problems, who had no hope of conceiving without assistance, believed they could increase their chances of assisted conception through actions like following dietary advice. This belief is important as the loss of control is considered a common experience in patients with infertility.

All this leads specialists to respond to the needs of patients in terms of practical information and online support, protecting them from the elements of greater exploitation to which they are vulnerable. They also need to meet the needs of those who have been advised to make lifestyle changes but are unable to do so, perhaps by offering more active dietary advice or encouraging them to accept the most suitable counseling. Women especially may feel a double failure if neither weight loss nor conception materializes and they are not willing to consider other ways to achieve pregnancy. Similarly, those who change lifestyle and continue to fail to conceive might need psychosexual help to adapt and still plan a future together and not a "prolonged mourning." Since parenthood is seen as one of the main goals of life, failing to achieve it can lead to a perception of defeat, as happens with other important goals and to considering useless any other form of self-realization.

Perceiving the loss or reduction of the ability to achieve a significant social role (e.g., feeling inferior, rejected, unable to control oneself, or somehow inadequate compared to friends or family regarding parenthood) can promote the onset of perceptions of failure. Furthermore, internal self-criticism can also give rise to a sense of defeat, and some studies have shown that infertile patients tend to exhibit high levels of this psychological process [14]. Indeed, infertility is perceived as a low-control stress factor, and infertile couples may feel isolated, stigmatized, or inadequate compared to their social networks.

Society may fail to recognize the pain caused by infertility, which can lead those struggling with it to hide their feelings. Previous research emphasizes that infertile people have deficiencies in fertility care regarding continuity of care and social support. Social media can provide social and psychological support to infertile people. Finding others who are experiencing similar experiences can lead to the realization that the person is not alone and that their feelings are reasonable. The research goal of Sormunen et al. [15] was to explore the role of social media for people affected by infertility. To collect the data, a computer-assisted, self-administered online cross-sectional questionnaire containing both open and closed questions was used. The questionnaire was linked to the bulletin board of six social forums on infertility. Both quantitative and qualitative analysis methods were used. A total of 132 participants completed the questionnaire, which contained questions about their use of social media to cope with infertility.

Results: Most of the questionnaires were answered by women (97.7%) via Facebook (87%). Over 60% of respondents had taken part in discussions about infertility on social media, over a period of 1–3 years; 39% had participated more than once a day. Half of the participants dedicated 1–3 h weekly to the forums and wrote one to five messages per week. The forums offered participants' information, solidarity, and the opportunity to receive and give support. However, a negative aspect described was advice that was not based on evidence. Infertility was experienced as an alienation from social life and a fragmentation as a person.

But there is more.

It is known that social support reduces stress and increases the quality of life of patients undergoing in vitro fertilization. The increase in the use of social media introduces a social support mechanism, but data regarding the effect of this support on the results of in vitro fertilization are scarce. The observational and retrospective study of Miller et al. [16] included women undergoing their first cycle of in vitro fertilization at a tertiary university medical center. Fertility outcomes were compared between 82 women who were active social media users (posting on Facebook at least 3 times a week) and 83 women who did not use Facebook or any other social media platform (the control group). For the social media group, all Facebook feed activities (Posts, Comments, Likes) for each participant were coded up to 8 weeks before the beta hCG test.

Social support was measured based on the average of "Likes" and "Comments" per post, on fertility outcomes. The social media group included more single women compared to the control group (17% vs. 5%, respectively, $p = 0.012$) and had a shorter duration of infertility. A trend in fertilization rates was found between the groups (social media group 58% compared to controls 50%, $p = 0.07$). No difference was found regarding the pregnancy rate between the groups ($p = 0.587$) compared to the controls (6% vs. 25%, $p = 0.042$). It emerged that social support (via Facebook) can have a positive effect on the outcomes of in vitro fertilization, particularly in terms of the abortion rate. Therefore, encouraging women to be active on Facebook during treatment, including OPU Day, can influence the results of the treatment itself.

And the men? The team led by Kruglova et al. [17] developed a mobile health app (mHealth app), Infotility XY, to promote male reproductive health. This study evaluated whether the use of the app led to greater knowledge of infertility risk factors and whether the change in knowledge was associated with the sociodemographic characteristics of the participants and/or the use of the app.

Participants were recruited between August and October 2020. Eligibility criteria included: identified as male, 18–45 years old, childless, no history of infertility, able to read and write in English/French, and had access to the Internet. Participants' fertility knowledge was assessed before and after using the app. App usage data were collected during the 2-week intervention period. The sample included 49 men aged between 18 and 45 years. Seventy-eight percent of participants had not previously sought information on fertility. Participants viewed, on average, 75% of the app's articles and 96% of participants stated that the app has increased their knowledge of fertility. Before using the app, 55% of men claimed to be aware of infertility risk factors, compared to 96% after using the app. This study provides evidence of the feasibility of an mHealth app to improve men's awareness of infertility risk factors. Given the positive relationship between male reproductive health and general health, greater awareness of infertility risk factors can lead to an improvement in men's overall health.

The study by Hanna and Gough [18] provided insights into men's narratives about infertility in the context of their intimate relationships. Clinical experience shows that infertility can have an impact on intimate relationships with the partner (both positively and negatively), but there is a scarcity of research on how men talk about such relational impacts and how they share their stories with other men. Men are often seen as the silent support partner in infertility contexts, with women portrayed as if they bear the weight of the relationship. The study was based on data from an online discussion forum for men only.

Results: Men's posts show that infertility tests relationships and that men use the surveilled forum to offer each other advice on how to deal with infertility in their relationships. Men have highlighted the feeling of having less agency compared to their partners in relation to infertility and consequently being less able to access support for themselves. This once again shows that the consideration of both individuals in infertile couples is very important to support relationships during any process of diagnosis and treatment for infertility.

Furthermore, the study by Woodard et al. [19] aimed to field test *Pathways*: a patient decision aid website for fertility preservation for young women affected by cancer. Doctors and computer technicians designed and optimized the "Pathways" patient website through four iterative cycles of review with doctors. Field tests evaluated the scores of the Fertility Preservation Knowledge Scale, the quality of women's decision-making features during use of the website, and the acceptance ratings of the website. Recruited patients achieved an average of 8.2 out of 13 (SD 1.6) on the fertility preservation knowledge scale. They rated genetic screening and having a biological child as decisive factors in their decision-making process and 71% indicated a preference for egg freezing. Most women (>85%) rated "Pathways" positively and all women (100%) stated they would recommend it to other women.

Another study by Gabarron et al. [20] analyzed the characteristics of posts shared over a 3-year period on three social media channels for diabetes (Facebook, Twitter, and Instagram) and user engagement (Likes, Comments, and Shares). All social media posts published by the Norwegian Diabetes Association between January 1, 2017 and December 31, 2019 were extracted. Two independent reviewers classified the posts into seven categories based on their content.

Results: A total of 1449 messages were posted. Posts of interviews and personal stories received 111% more Likes, 106% more Comments, and 112% more Shares than miscellaneous posts (all $p < 0.001$). Messages posted about awareness days and other celebrations were 41% more likely to receive Likes than miscellaneous posts ($p < 0.001$). Conversely, posts on research and innovation received 31% fewer Likes ($p < 0.001$), 35% fewer Comments ($p = 0.02$), and 25% fewer Shares ($p = 0.03$) than miscellaneous posts. Health education posts received 38% fewer Comments ($p = 0.003$) but were shared 39% more than miscellaneous posts ($p = 0.007$). With regard to social media channels, Facebook and Instagram posts were both 35 times more likely than Twitter posts to receive Likes, and 60 times and almost 10 times more likely to receive Comments, respectively ($p < 0.001$). Compared to text-only posts, those with videos had 3 times greater chance of receiving Likes, an almost 4 times greater chance of receiving Comments, and a 2.5 times greater chance of being shared (all $p < 0.001$). Including both videos and emoji in posts increased the chances of receiving Likes by almost 7 times ($p < 0.001$). Adding an emoji to posts increased their chances of receiving Likes and being shared by 71% and 144%, respectively ($p < 0.001$). This led to a better understanding of infertility and sexual dysfunctions resulting from diabetes.

From the discussions reviewed on Twitter, the study by Balasubramanian et al. [21] evaluated content focused on male infertility using the official Urology Ontology hashtag, #MaleInfertility. Symplur, a Twitter analysis service, was used to analyze the activity, users, and content of tweets related to #MaleInfertility between August 2015 and November 2018. Activity was quantified based on monthly tweets and cumulative annual users. Users were classified based on geographical location, occupation, and organizational affiliation. Content analysis was performed by analyzing retweets, links, media, mentions, responses, frequently used words, and hashtags.

Results: A total of 11,325 tweets and 3241 users using the hashtag #MaleInfertility were identified. Most of the tweets (73%) were sent with links. The average ± SD number of #MaleInfertility tweets per month increased from 152 ± 47 in 2015 to 439 ± 2013 in 2018 ($p < 0.001$). During this period, the number of users increased from 95 to 3241. Linear regression revealed that the discussion on #MaleInfertility increased by 8.7 tweets per month and 80 users per month during the study period ($p < 0.0001$). Users tweeted from 22 countries and doctors made up 39% of the top 100 influencers. The most popular associated hashtags included #Infertility, #IVF, and #Sperm. Content coding of tweets revealed that tweets were primarily focused on providing online support to patients. In conclusion: video streaming. Over 30 million visitors per day seek health information on the YouTube platform. Videos related to men's health have proliferated immensely, but content produced by qualified health professionals remains scarce. In fact, the study by Zaila et al. [22] analyzed educational streaming videos on YouTube created in collaboration with a large university health system focused on male infertility, men's health, and Peyronie's disease, uploaded between 2016 and 2018. All videos featured a certified urologist with training in andrology. Using YouTube's native analysis tools, data on views, engagement, and geographical coverage were extrapolated until 8/2019. Data were obtained for streaming videos on male infertility ($n = 3$), general men's health ($n = 2$), and Peyronie's disease ($n = 1$). Video duration ranged from 29 to 51 minutes, with an average video duration of 39 minutes and 41 seconds. The average actual viewing time by viewers ranged from 3:45 to 8:30. The total number of views was 646,684, with a viewing time of nearly 3 million minutes, reaching viewers in 47 countries. Fifty-three percent of the viewing time occurred on a mobile device and 33% on a personal computer. Among these, the video "Movember and why you should support men's health" was part of an educational campaign and did not receive as many overall views as the other five videos. A recent study by Warren et al. [23] has shown that YouTube videos featuring doctors were of significantly higher quality and less distorted, but had fewer views compared to videos that did not feature a doctor.

15.2 Conclusion

Despite the growing demand for information and strategies to prevent infertility, many couples decide to stop treatments even without achieving a pregnancy. The internet was also helpful for the study by Marcus et al. [24]. Registered users were recruited from an independent infertility website and asked to complete a structured questionnaire. Eighty users completed the questionnaire. Fifty-eight percent of patients received treatment at a single center and 78% paid for the treatment themselves. Forty-two percent of couples intended to undergo only one treatment cycle and 60% reported undergoing more cycles than originally planned. Ten percent of patients regretted not stopping treatment earlier. The most common reasons patients opted against further treatment cycles were financial constraints (46%), emotional burden (35%), poor response to treatment (29%), and poor egg quality (19%). This shows that the decision to undertake or stop treatment is a difficult process that exclusively involves the couple. Medical results, although always evolving, cannot deny that the relational structure of couples, quality of life, social network, and emotional potential are the prerequisites conditioning the desire for parenthood. Much more needs to be done in strengthening systemic teams and balancing scientific factors and psychosexual factors, starting with basic training that should teach practitioners to see healthcare as a system of specialists who build "ad hoc" health projects for each individual infertile couple.

References

1. Dube L, Nkosi-Mafutha N, Balsom AA, Gordon JL (2021) Infertility-related distress and clinical targets for psychotherapy: a qualitative study. BMJ Open 11(11):e050373. https://doi.org/10.1136/bmjopen-2021-050373s
2. Martins MV, Peterson BD, Almeida V, Mesquita-Guimarães J, Costa ME (2014) Dyadic dynamics of perceived social support in couples facing infertility. Hum Reprod 29(1):83–89. https://doi.org/10.1093/humrep/det403. PMID: 24218401
3. Frick-Bruder V (1919) Couple relationship and couple dynamics of sterile marriages. Arch Gynecol Obstet 245(1–4):1050–1052. German. PMID: 2802684. https://doi.org/10.1007/BF02417680
4. Walen HR, Lachman ME (2000) Social support and strain from partner, family, and friends: costs and benefits for men and women in adulthood. J Soc Pers Relat 17(1):5–30
5. Lund R, Sejbaek CS, Christensen U, Schmidt L (2009) The impact of social relations on the incidence of severe depressive symptoms among infertile women and men. Hum Reprod 24(11):2810–2820. https://doi.org/10.1093/humrep/dep257
6. Greil AL, Slauson-Blevins K, McQuillan J (2010) The experience of infertility: a review of recent literature. Sociol Health Illn 32(1):140–162. https://doi.org/10.1111/j.1467-9566.2009.01213.x
7. Torrent-Sellens J, Díaz-Chao Á, Soler-Ramos I, Saigí-Rubió F (2016) Journal of medical internet research. JMIR Publications, Toronto. Modeling and predicting eHealth usage in Europe: a multidimensional approach from an online survey conducted on 13,000 European Union Internet users
8. Wingert S, Harvey CDH, Duncan KA, Berry RE (2005) Assessing the needs of assisted reproductive technology users of an online bulletin board. Int J Consumer Stud 29:468–478
9. Cousineau TM, Lord SE, Seibring AR, Corsini EA, Viders JC, Lakhani SR (2004) A multimedia psychosocial support program for couples receiving infertility treatment: a feasibility study. Fertil Steril 81(3):532–538. https://doi.org/10.1016/j.fertnstert.2003.08.021
10. Weissmann A, Gotlieb L, Ward S, Greenblatt E, Casper RF (2000) Use of the internet by infertile couples. Fertil Steril 73(6):1179–1182. https://doi.org/10.1016/s0015-0282(00)00515-x
11. Huang JY, Al-Fozan H, Tan SL, Tulandi T (2003) Internet use by patients seeking infertility treatment. Int J Gynaecol Obstet 83(1):75–76. https://doi.org/10.1016/s0020-7292(03)00253-4
12. Himmel W, Meyer J, Kochen MM, Michelmann HW (2005) Information needs and visitors' experience of an Internet expert forum on infertility. J Med Internet Res 7(2):e20. https://doi.org/10.2196/jmir.7.2.e20

13. Tennen H, Affleck G, Mendola R (1991) Causal explanations for infertility: their relation to control appraisals and psychological adjustment. In: Stanton AL, Dunkel-Schetter C (eds) Infertility: perspectives from stress and coping research. Plenum Press, London, pp 109–131. https://doi.org/10.1007/978-1-4899-0753-0_6
14. Cugino TM (2007) Psychological impact of infertility. Best Pract Res Clin Obstet Gynaecol 21:293–308
15. Sormunen T, Karlgren K, Aanesen A, Fossum B, Westerbotn M (2020) The role of social media for persons affected by infertility. BMC Womens Health 20(1):112. https://doi.org/10.1186/s12905-020-00964-0
16. Miller N, Pundak C, Cohen G, Issakov G, Gluska H, Gandelsman E, Frishman EK, David L, Bookstein SP, Goldenberg J, Wiser A (2022) Can social support on Facebook influence fertility outcomes? Reprod Sci 29(1):212–219. https://doi.org/10.1007/s43032-021-00611-5. Epub 2021 May 18. PMID: 34008155
17. Kruglova K, Gelgoot EN, Chan P, Lo K, Rosberger Z, Bélanger E, Kazdan J, Robins S, Zelkowitz P (2021) Risky business: increasing fertility knowledge of men in the general public using the mobile health application *Infotility XY*. Am J Mens Health 15(5):15579883211049027. https://doi.org/10.1177/15579883211049027
18. Hanna E, Gough B (2017) Men's accounts of infertility within their intimate partner relationships: an analysis of online forum discussions. J Reprod Infant Psychol 35(2):150–158. https://doi.org/10.1080/02646838.2017.1278749. Epub 2017 Jan 19. PMID: 29517356
19. Woodard TL, Hoffman AS, Covarrubias LA, Holman D, Schover L, Bradford A, Hoffman DB, Mathur A, Thomas J, Volk RJ (2018) The pathways fertility preservation decision aid website for women with cancer: development and field testing. J Cancer Surviv 12(1):101–114. https://doi.org/10.1007/s11764-017-0649-5. Epub 2017 Oct 15. PMID: 29034438
20. Gabarron E, Larbi D, Dorronzoro E, Hasvold PE, Wynn R, Årsand E (2020) Factors engaging users of diabetes social media channels on Facebook, Twitter, and Instagram: observational study. J Med Internet Res 22(9):e21204. https://doi.org/10.2196/21204
21. Balasubramanian A, Yu J, Thirumavalavan N, Lipshultz LI, Hotaling JM, Pastuszak AW (2020) Analyzing online Twitter discussion for male infertility via the hashtag #MaleInfertility. Urol Pract 7(1):68–74. https://doi.org/10.1097/UPJ.0000000000000066. Epub 2019 May 7. PMID: 37317387
22. Zaila KE, Osadchiy V, Anderson AS, Eleswarapu SV, Mills JN (2020) Popularity and worldwide reach of targeted, evidence-based internet streaming video interventions focused on men's health topics. Transl Androl Urol 9(3):1374–1381. https://doi.org/10.21037/tau-20-580
23. Warren C, Shah T, Ward B et al (2020) 184 evaluation of YouTube videos on male hypogonadism. J Sex Med 17:S62. https://doi.org/10.1016/j.jsxm.2019.11.130
24. Marcus D, Marcus A, Johnson A, Marcus S (2011) Infertility treatment: when is it time to give up? An Internet-based survey. Hum Fertil (Camb) 14(1):29–34. https://doi.org/10.3109/14647273.2010.541971. PMID: 21329471

Chapter 16
Individuals, Couples, and Families: Clinical Cases

No one better than an infertile couple can describe the unique situation at the base of the desire for a child and the will to undertake an assisted medical procedure. Each individual within the two-person story has "a family history, a personal clinical and emotional experience, as well as a baggage of social relationships." With this are associated the experiences of the previous relational stories of the individuals and the story of the couple. Here are some stories.

16.1 Luisa and Gianluca

Luisa is a Kindergarten teacher, 34 years old, and Gianluca is a 38-year-old engineer. They have been married for 2 years, but have known each other for 5 years.

16.2 Gianluca

Gianluca arrives for the first psychosexual visit, referred by the andrologist of our IRCCS San Raffaele Sexual Medicine Center in Milan (Italy), with orgasmic dysfunction and anejaculation (inability to ejaculate). He says that the symptom appeared immediately after the wedding and that it is becoming an element of inadequacy and conflict with Luisa, because they would like to have a child. Both are natives of Southern Italy and the local culture cannot conceive of a couple without children.

He also reports that he would have liked the cause of his dysfunction to be organic and not psychosexual.

In response to my acknowledgment that it is human to believe that one can control everything in life, he nods and shows deep sadness.

E. V. Longhi, *Framing Sexual Dysfunctions and Diseases during Fertility Treatment*, https://doi.org/10.1007/978-3-031-76726-5_16

During the sexual anamnesis, it emerges that Gianluca has had sexual intercourse only with paid partners and does not have an experience of sexual intercourse other than in a passive role. Luisa's patience has made him gain courage in affection and passion, but he has never experienced a complete sexual relationship.

To this is added the fact that at that time Gianluca describes himself as very worried about his mother who has been diagnosed with breast cancer. "My father is not able to handle the situation and my sister works in Canada." Gianluca complains and plans to move his mother to Milan, his city of residence.

To my question "How do you think you will manage your mother and at the same time undertake a psychosexual path? And… assisted reproduction?" Gianluca shakes his head and answers me "I don't know, but I have no alternatives." Reassured about the various procedures that will however have distinct times, I reiterate that, if he allows me, he and his wife will be looked after and will not be alone. I then ask for an individual meeting with his wife and then one as a couple.

16.3 Luisa

Luisa arrives at the meeting displaying an enterprising character and full of resolutive hopes. "I was hoping you would invite me doctor" she begins and smiling I clarify to her that it is not only my professional methodology, but that I need useful information from both members of the couple. Luisa is very satisfied with her work and complains about Gianluca's excessive rationality, working even in the evening and on weekends.

Her parents are healthy and she has two younger sisters to whom she is very attached and who still live at home. She did not have significant relationships before Gianluca, in part because she had enlisted in the Carabinieri for 6 years. She decided to leave the Force due to the concerns expressed by her parents because they viewed her life as being in danger and because her grandfather (her mother's father), a carabiniere, had died in service at the age of 45.

Being a mother for Luisa is an important and fulfilling experience "Children cheer me up and are full of surprises." Unlike Gianluca, Luisa reports having had sporadic but satisfying sexual relationships with partners who had not shown sexual dysfunctions.

Yet she is very concerned about her husband's sexuality because she sees he is disappointed, guilty for not making her happy and she admits that it was she who convinced Gianluca to consult an andrologist.

16.4 The Medical Team

In communications with the andrologist and geneticists, I ask to respect the couple's timing and to share a time-based project with sex therapy as a priority and then the evaluation of a parenting project. In the meantime, through a spermogram, Gianluca is found to be oligospermic and begins an andrological fertility therapy to improve the spermatic picture.

16.5 The Couple

Sexological consultations are scheduled every 2 weeks, so that the couple can apply the exercises I proposed.

The perseverance in performing them has been subject to alternating events. Sometimes due to Gianluca's excessive work, sometimes due to the stress that the couple was experiencing on this journey. For this purpose, periods of "only play" between the parties (without exercises) were scheduled so that the couple could catch their breath.

Given the nature of Gianluca's dysfunction, results came about where occasionally ejaculation was missing "You're right, I did it my way. I didn't do your exercise doctor and I didn't go further." Gianluca apologized when necessary, because joking about his excess of control, he could count on my "thank goodness even you Doctor, are human sometimes too."

A lot of stress and anxiety also came from the fact that the sperm levels were not improving as much as expected. Gianluca showed a burst of responsibility: he started physical exercise, and proposed a more regulated diet and all this led the couple to three attempts at assisted procreation.

Luisa produced few eggs and the couple's anxieties multiplied: She started a yoga course, took a period of leave from work, and enrolled in autogenic training courses.

On the third attempt came the pregnancy, not without anxieties, nausea, and panic attacks. In the end, Andrea was born.

16.6 The Team

In all phases of the couple's relationship, the psychosexologist was always present: as a liaison with the other doctors and as a liaison between the spouses and the family of origin of both. Gianluca's mother underwent a quadrantectomy, fortunately without further adjuvant therapies. However, the period of cohabitation with the mother-in-law, the guest of the couple, before and after the operation, during the second month of Luisa's pregnancy was difficult. "I felt suffocated with my mother-in-law who was calling her son every minute because she couldn't manage alone at home. I was alone, Gianluca came back from work late in the evening and on weekends he divided his time between his mother and me. The couple had disappeared. When my mother-in-law returned home, I had panic attacks because I was alone for almost the whole day and I asked my mother to come and keep me company."

The talks with the sexologist continued in each of these relational phases, online. After Andrea's birth, the couple asked to be followed up for a discussion. For a year, the time to return as a couple, with an active sexuality, and with other life projects.

16.7 Francesca and Arturo

Our IRCCS Birth Center refers Arturo (45 years old) to me, because for a few months he has been experiencing erectile dysfunction and hypoactive desire during intercourse. They started an assisted fertilization program a few weeks ago.

16.8 Arturo

He comes with Francesca (39 years old): they have been married for 5 years and have known each other for 7 years. They describe their marriage as "uphill": a month before the wedding, Francesca's father dies of a heart attack and three women are left alone, her mother, sister, and the patient.

"Three women without a guide" Arturo reports, so they kept the wedding date because "a male figure of reference and support would enter the family." On the wedding day, Francesca reports being approached by Arturo's sister who confided in her "you'll see what you're getting."

On the wedding night, Arturo was admitted for symptoms of anxiety–depression. He was hospitalized for 3 days and discharged with appropriate therapy. Until this point, Arturo had shared Francesca's description in the interviews, then the conflict exploded before my eyes.

They did not go on honeymoon, waiting instead for Arturo to recover, Francesca reports in tears, "because I saw a new suffering in front of me."

The husband resentfully denies any kind of suffering on the part of his wife and maintains that Francesca, under the shadow of the father, had a fight with the sister-in-law and that her family sided against him.

In the meantime, Francesca and Arturo live through periods of continuous confrontations and bulimic attacks with the result that their weight increased by about 10 kg.

16.9 The Team

I shared with the geneticists and the andrologist (who had started following Arturo) the fact that we were facing a relational conflict and that the discussion of sexuality would come as a consequence. During the interviews with the couple, Arturo was convinced that he needed a male interlocutor in the form of a psychiatrist, with whom to share the pharmacological therapy and a robust confrontation. I also spoke with the psychiatrist several times and shared with the rest of the team the ongoing process.

16.10 Francesca

When the relationship seemed more conciliatory and less conflictual, Francesca, unable to follow a diet that would allow her to lose weight (and be able to invest in a possible pregnancy), decided on a gastric reduction surgery that had more than a few consequences.

"Sometimes I can't resist and I drink fizzy drinks…then I keep vomiting, I can't stand up and Artuto gets worried, slams the front door and stays out for hours." Despite these difficulties, the psychosexual interviews also lead to a rapprochement of the couple. Arturo manages to have decent sperm levels and the process for assisted fertilization begins.

16.11 The Couple

Two attempts promoted by the geneticists with a result of twin birth: Livio and Rossana. During the pregnancy, Francesca, despite having lost 15 kg, from the third month of the pregnancy remained in bed. She asked for leave from work (company secretary) and Arturo continued his professional activity at an International Company.

Everything seemed calmer, when Arturo lost his job because "my managerial position was eliminated." The situation became more complex: Francesca tried to be understanding with her husband, but concern for the future prevailed.

Arturo changed psychiatrists because "that one (the psychiatrist) doesn't talk, he only gives drugs and I don't need them." His sister made it clear immediately "don't ask for help from us (sister and mother). Now you have a wife, you can sort it out for yourself." On Francesca's side, her mother advised her to move into the parental home to be cared for and to be comfortable.

"I would gladly do it" the partner confided to me "but I'm afraid that Arturo will make a scene and I fear that he won't tolerate my absence."

A new couple's program was set up where Arturo had to take care of the legal and administrative part of the professional situation (and be relieved from assisting his wife) and Francesca was to be looked after for a few hours a day by mutual friends, which was appreciated by Arturo.

Francesca's mother, with whom supportive talks were held, was asked to be present through phone calls and little messages.

16.12 The Team

The birth arrived. The little ones were born healthy and full of life. Arturo seemed to be healed on the spot and so did Francesca. However, Arturo's work problems took over, he continued to see the psychiatrist and the labor law attorney he had entrusted himself to. I arranged a series of more intense meetings between the psychiatrist Arturo because, as his sister said, "he was not a man with broad shoulders."

Francesca's mother had the opportunity to step in during the breastfeeding and weaning of the little ones. The meetings with me continued for a few months, until the couple understood that it was better to "separate" as spouses, while continuing to share parenthood. Arturo found work after 2 years and, once the marital home was sold, Francesca found an apartment near her mother and sisters. Now the little ones see their father twice a week and on alternate weekends.

16.13 Stefano and Marta

Stefano and Marta are a couple in life and in profession: they are both lawyers and work in the same firm, which Stefano's father left to his only son. Marta has a brother "very different from me, he seems like a tourist in life. He only does what his wife tells him, except in his profession (lawyer)."

Stefano teaches at the University in Bologna and Marta was one of his students. They have a 15-year age difference. "I would never have married a peer because I find them superficial," explains Marta immediately, presenting herself as controlled, not inclined to express emotionality, and with a very severe critical judgment.

Stefano appears to be a calm person more ready to be the "guardian" of his wife than the husband.

They have been married for 2 years with the blessing of their families of origin even though a dear friend of Marta seems to have warned her "you'll end up being your husband's nurse."

The "casus belli" of the psychosexual consultation was that Marta's brother became a father a year after the wedding and she thought "how can it be that a superficial person like my brother has a child almost without thinking about it and I, who have always deserved everything, have not yet succeeded?"

The couple has already turned to a Fertility Center that has diagnosed "idiopathic infertility."

For Marta it is difficult to accept such a "sentence" because "I'm not crazy and I have no problems, why resort to a psychosexual therapist?"

Stefano, on the other hand, reports feeling absolved because his own virility is not the cause of problems and neither is his wife's biological femininity.

16.14 The Team

In agreement with the geneticists and psychologists of the Center, a psychosexual path is started because from the anamnesis it emerges that the couple sustain an effusive sexuality, neither passionate nor erotic, because these components are experienced as "violence and aggression."

16.15 The Couple

At the beginning, Marta is hesitant and not inclined to express anger, resentment, and suffering toward her brother and the stalemate of the couple. The question that turned out to be a turning point was "what could happen if the child does not arrive?"

For Marta it was impossible to hypothesize such an ending "Why are you asking me? Do you think I'm not capable?" The psychosexual therapists, I explain, often have to assume uncomfortable and unpopular roles: "The couple has all the resources to do well even while contemplating other projects for the future, so as not to be unprepared."

Stefano shows surprise and confesses "I never even imagined it, why didn't I think about it?"

The desires of every couple are often omnipotent and Marta receives the message beginning "I'm not weak, but I always have to emancipate myself from someone. I hoped that Stefano would solve everything and today I find myself in a situation that I had not foreseen. He also needs me."

The family stories clarified other family myths.

On Marta's part "my parents taught me that affections are earned and I have never caused problems. It was impossible to tell them "I'm scared, I can't do it" because my brother has always been the baby of the family, who had to be understood and helped. A big egoist. I had to be the one who succeeded and did everything by herself…."

On Stefano's part the situation was still unclear. The son of separated parents, he reports of his mother's sunny disposition, full of interests, who decided on separation to reclaim her own life.

Stefano's father belongs to an ancient noble Sicilian family that still lives today as a chosen caste. Despite having given the practice to his son he does not fail to remark "you are a niggardly son. You kicked me out of my practice. You are ungrateful and I am very disappointed by your behavior."

Stefano at the time of the consultation decided to cut off any type of relationship with his father but talks about him continuously.

It is clear that suffering for the couple is one of the bonds of attention, protection, and care for two to redeem "the previous life of children" as Marta defines it.

In subsequent interviews, Marta is given the opportunity to present herself or to be absent so as not to enter into symmetry with her defensive rigidities.

From that moment she appears more participatory and, in the case of absence from the interviews, she reports to her husband what she would have said in the session, as per my instructions.

Just before embarking on the assisted fertilization journey, Stefano confides in me that Marta during the day says "we have to tell this to the doctor and you ask her for advice."

We work on different levels: the relationship with the families of origin, Stefano's role of husband and "temporary guardian," Marta's alexithymia (the inability to express feelings), the couple's plans for the future with or without children, and sexuality.

16.16 The Team

Following the first attempt at assisted fertilization (after a year of psychosexual interviews), Francesco arrives, the name of the paternal grandfather.

At Francesco's baptism, even the Sicilian grandfather is present and he hugs Stefano for the first time telling him "thank you for making me a grandfather and also, before that, a father."

Stefano asked to continue the interviews alone for a few months, then it was my task to discharge him, because he could now do without everyone, except for his family.

16.17 Massimo and Clara

They come to my attention of their own volition because they are about to embark on a journey of assisted fertilization in great secrecy. They have been married for 6 years and Clara has always been Massimo's best friend. They both work: Massimo in a Travel Agency and Clara has a hairdressing business.

16.18 The Previous Story

They describe their sexuality as good and satisfying. Massimo underwent a penile prosthesis operation 3 years ago. Eight years earlier he was the victim of a trauma that significantly affected their life.

During a storm, Massimo and Clara, coming out of the Cinema, seek shelter, but while running, a tree breaks and falls on Massimo's back. "I couldn't feel my body, I was completely paralyzed, Clara was screaming and a passerby, I still bless him to this day, called an ambulance. I found myself in a wheelchair, myelopathic."

Clara, due to the traumatic stress, began to suffer from insomnia, sleepwalking, and nightmares.

"They were hard years of rehabilitation and psychiatrists because my mood was not so high. I felt lost and I even challenged Clara, telling her that I didn't love her and that she deserved much more than a cripple," confesses Massimo.

They did not see each other for a year, during which time each of them followed an individual therapeutic path.

Then, through a mutual friend, they met again at a Birthday party and from there they started dating again. "I never stopped thinking about him and it hurt me when he pushed me away or told me that I deserved a normal guy," emphasizes Clara.

The year before getting married, an andrologist proposed to Massimo the implantation of a penile prosthesis to have a sexuality like all young people of their age (30 years old). After the intervention and adequate clinical support, Massimo and Marta rediscovered a satisfying sexuality, albeit with much fear of not being able to make it.

And now that life is smiling at them, they want to go further. A child.

Based on past experience where their families of origin had opposed the prosthetic surgery, they want to share their "desire only with a professional, under secrecy."

16.19 The Team

Faced with this eventuality, I speak with the andrologist who implanted the penile prosthesis, asking him if Massimo had proceeded with cryopreservation and unfortunately the answer was negative.

I begged the andrologist to be present at a meeting with the couple and after some resistance we agreed on this.

I told the couple that I needed to confront the andrologist they had turned to because I needed information in their presence.

"There is no problem" was Massimo's impulsive response. Clara seemed more hesitant: "what worries you doctor?" "Nothing dear, I just need information beyond yours to understand how to help you best."

It was not easy to set up the meeting. The andrologist brought the result of Massimo's spermogram before the prosthetic intervention. The sperm levels were far below the norm and for this reason he did not recommend cryopreservation.

16.20 The Couple

Massimo's reaction was one of anger and betrayal toward the andrologist and doctors in general. Clara was almost relieved. In subsequent talks, Clara clarified that the idea of a child fascinated her but she realized that there would be no room for a little one.

Massimo occupied all the non-work time: although he was autonomous in daily practical activities, he showed an infantile fragility "He needs attention, appreciation and often falls asleep hugging me." Clara needed a partner, not a child and Massimo made her feel useful, necessary, and important.

It took time to share with Massimo that his tenacity had rewarded him in being a well-liked professional, with many friends, and a wife who loved him and did not pity him. It was shared with the couple that Massimo needed to relate to children to understand how much his desire for a child was a way to prove he was like his friends or was really a desire for fatherhood.

They volunteered in a "family home." After three Sundays in that context for a couple of hours each time, Massimo wrote to me "better that I am the child of the family…".

16.21 Giulio and Federica

The couple asks for a psychosexual consultation and is sent by the Department of Gynecology. Giulio, 42 years old, an accountant, and Federica, a general surgery doctor, have been married for 4 years and their sexual relations appear painful, sporadic, and at the initiative of the husband.

16.22 Federica

She has been suffering from endometriosis for 8 years and has also undergone laparoscopic surgery but "the suffering and pain are continuous, even while I work or talk to patients." She had a previous marriage, which lasted 6 months, until she realized that her ex-husband was gambling considerable sums. The daughter of doctors "I couldn't risk a life with an unreliable man and my family made me pay for it. We were on everyone's lips, and my father, a renowned surgeon, suffered from the ironic and sarcastic comments of some colleagues." Despite this, Federica is on the rise "and is more married to the Hospital than to me," jokes Giulio. She has an older brother with whom she has a stable relationship but the real bond is with her mother.

16.23 Giulio

He has a younger brother who works in import/export, he married an Asian woman, and lives in Shanghai. He has no children. Before meeting Federica, he reports having had two important relationships with a satisfying sexuality.

The previous stories ended through his own choice because he did not feel ready for marriage and a family. The son of separated parents, the father lives in Venice and is retired, the mother, a painter, lives in Milan, like Giulio. He sees her every week (the mother): she is cared for by a caregiver because a few months ago she received a diagnosis of Parkinson's. Giulio talks about it with great suffering and feels alone in this situation "Federica is nice, she gives me medical advice, my brother calls every ten days, but my mother only sees me and her friends. Even the gallery owners (with whom she has worked for 40 years) are moving away…and my mother suffers in silence." Seeing therefore, Federica, always suffering and nervous "is a great pain for me, we are a couple of 'friends'. If I approach her she tells me that I suffocate her and intimacy is always an obstacle race."

16.24 The Couple

They regularly attend the interviews and Federica always speaks with a professional tone and little empathy. She does not love her own body and would like Giulio to understand not to touch her, not to hug her, not to seek tenderness. She has no sexual experience with her husband and reports that if she could she would do without sexuality, but she wants a child.

She has decided on assisted fertilization even though the chances of success will be slim. Giulio reflects that a child would be for him a way to invest a part of the tenderness that he cannot share with his wife.

During the interviews, I increasingly get the feeling that the couple is made up of "two forever children": every Sunday they go to lunch at her parents' and Federica calls her mother three times a day. In the evening, Federica "still works—Giulio reports—she sits in front of the computer, writes scientific articles, prepares the slides for the Congresses." Giulio reads, watches television, and hopes every night to be able to sleep in her arms.

16.25 The Team

Talking with the reference gynecologists, we agree that Federica is purely "a doctor" and not inclined to lose control of the role. We reflect on how ready she would be to accept a failure in the fertilization attempt, how much Giulio would be even more submissive to his wife's emotions and how the couple's relationship could change. A joint meeting is decided: the couple, the reference gynecologists, Giulio's andrologist, and me.

16.26 The Couple

From the start the meeting took on a style of "confrontation between doctors" and it was not easy to loosen the scientific tone, introducing more reflections on the couple's balances, on the emotions of both and on the alternative planning to achieve parenthood.

Giulio in the end put himself in a mediating position with Federica trying to reflect on other opportunities, even as a couple, hypothesizing projects for the future. Federica was unyielding in her decision.

Shortly thereafter, the couple informed me that they had turned to another Center for Gynecology and Obstetrics. The discussions continued as a couple and individually, especially with Giulio: his mother continued to worsen and even the caregiver reported often finding herself in difficulty due to the lady's aggressive behavior. Until one day she mistook Giulio for her husband "what are you doing here? You've remarried. Go to your new wife!" What happened was mortifying for Giulio ("I feel like an orphan now"). Nevertheless, he accompanied his mother to specialist visits and screenings.

Federica's family, for their part, brought all the medical knowledge they had to bear and in the end there were three attempts at assisted fertilization and three failures.

Federica reacted first with disappointment, anger, and suffering and then, regaining control of her role, she began to belittle her husband "You always think about hugs like a child…I married a worthless man. Imagine if you had become a father …".

In the meantime, Giulio lost his mother, his brother returned for a few weeks with his wife to Italy. The latter decided after a few days to return to Shanghai because she did not get along with her sister-in-law (Federica) and with Italian customs. There were also two meetings with Giulio and his brother: they talked about their mother, the suffering of the moment, and the absence of their respective wives.

When the brother returned to Shanghai, Giulio felt alone: he went to visit his father and saw "an old man who lived among books, paintings and exhibitions: with a second wife, a good and simple woman, who let him have his way." He felt doubly alone.

During the last meeting with the couple Federica and Giulio, they discussed the continuation of their marriage. Federica showed no doubts: they still had their profession and maybe a dog. Then came Biagio, a cheerful and affectionate Maltese. Giulio asked for more meetings: he got a promotion and moved to Berlin. "On weekends I return to Milan to see my friends and my wife, if she is not on duty at the Hospital. On the phone Federica is 'a sweetheart', and on weekends, apart from lunch with the in-laws, we see friends and we are fine." Giulio, unlike Federica, has kept in touch with me: every now and then he updates me on the news via SMS and especially sends me pictures of Biagio. "I love Federica very much, I would never leave her, but I only have you Doctor to talk to without being criticized … Who can understand me better? Let me know when you get tired of my messages…".

16.27 Alvise and Eden

The couple comes to my consultation on the referral of a colleague andrologist from a region in Central Italy. Alvise immediately reports that he has suffered from erectile dysfunction since his first sexual intercourse and Eden has difficulty with penetration (vaginismus). Sexual relations have become rare and they want a child. "The andrologist sent us to you because your Center is a place of excellence and the journey (to Milan) does not scare us." Alvise specifies and Eden nods in agreement. They are the same age, 39, and both work in the same pharmaceutical company: he as a warehouseman and she as a Secretary to Management.

16.28 Alvise

He begins by saying that he is of Venetian origins: his parents and his sister Lucinda, who is married with two children, and his maternal grandmother who lives with them, reside in Treviso. Alvise moved to Central Italy after marrying Eden, 5 years ago, and found work through his wife. He is bothered that his wife earns more than him and feels guilty when he buys anything for himself. Before Eden, he only had sexual relationships and met his wife through mutual friends. Alvise's family of origin, especially his mother and grandmother, suffered from his departure and for this reason he tries to return home every fortnight. This fact causes quite a few complaints from Eden's parents, who would like their daughter to always be on site. Not surprisingly, the in-laws live in the same building on the floor above the couple.

16.29 Eden

She appears to be a very calm, sweet woman, almost "resigned" to her parents' control. She reports that she was adopted at the age of 4, after her parents had lost a child to crib death.

Eden has no memories of her early years with her adoptive parents and reports that they have always given her everything: "my father always played with me, while my mother, a high school teacher, always followed my academic performance. They wanted me to go to university but once I got my accounting diploma. I decided to be independent and started working." First in the Administration of a Supermarket, then in her father's hardware store, then in the current Company. She had no significant relationships before marriage and no full sexual relationships except with her husband.

16.30 The Couple

Seeing them together, Alvise and Eden seem like two people with a great work ethic but with little ability to defend their intimacy. "I was not welcomed with great affection by my in-laws." Alvise confirms "My mother-in-law immediately told me that Eden deserved a better man and of a higher social status." The father-in-law was more welcoming but the atmosphere at home is determined by the mother-in-law "always on her high horse." Eden reports with irony.

Alvise's move was taken for granted by the in-laws who met the groom's parents only on the wedding day. Alvise's mother is worried about her son and welcomes Eden as a daughter. "My mother-in-law prepares the dishes I like the most, we go to the hairdresser together and often window shop," Eden says.

However, every time they return home from Treviso, the punishment arrives straight away. "What are you going to do with those 'peasants' (Alvise's parents own farms employing workers for the cultivation of cereals)? What's missing here? Did they at least give you something? Trips cost money."

In addition to this, every evening, returning from work, the in-laws enter the couple's house (they have a set of keys for security) to see if Alvise helps at home, if they have done the shopping, what they are cooking.

Not to mention the weekends "where I find them in our bedroom already at 7.00 in the morning because the father-in-law needs a hand in the store or in the garden," Alvise huffs.

Eden has a strong sense of guilt: she cannot react and does not rebel against her adoptive parents because "they lost a child before me, my mother abandoned me and I can't make them suffer." The only time Alvise tried to ask his in-laws for more privacy he was told "remember that you are in our house and you have a roof because we gave it to you."

16.31 The Therapeutic Team

Alvise's andrologist, having no tools to collaborate except pharmacological ones, gave me carte blanche. Alvise began to take every day a therapy for erectile dysfunction in great secrecy from both families of origin. I requested and obtained a meeting with Alvise's family online and they proved very collaborative. Especially, the 90-year-old grandmother who had even spoken with a priest for advice. Eden's family refused saying "their problems, we have done our part." This is because Eden had turned to the same gynecologist as the mother and no one kept the secret.

16.32 The Couple

Parallel to the sexual sphere, we began to put order in the relational life of the couple until Alvise and Eden looked for an apartment for rent on the other side of the city. It took them a while to look for it, furnish it, and in this Alvise's family was very generous.

In the meantime, on the sexual sphere, each of them had specific individual and couple exercises. On weekends, they safeguarded their privacy, locking the bedroom door, and started going out more often in the evening with friends "even just for a sandwich," confesses Alvise.

After about a year, with two meetings a month, sexuality began to be more satisfying and they moved into the new house. The in-laws were prepared little by little for the couple's house move, rationalizing it with the fact that Eden could not always stay "in the bell jar" overprotected and controlled in full view of parents. They agreed on a lunch or dinner a week at the in-laws even if they never understood this choice "you let yourself be manipulated by the first one to come along," scolded the mother "With all that your father and I have done for you."

Eden suffered a lot because of this reaction and it was difficult for her to consider the selfishness of the parents. Then came the umpteenth blackmail "since you want independence and want to mature, what are you waiting for to have a child?" Eden in the previous 6 months had two spontaneous abortions a few weeks into pregnancy and the new gynecologist (not the mother's) advised her to try assisted fertilization.

And here they are again in Milan. I followed them during the therapies, the screenings, and always without the in-laws knowing. Alvise's parents and even his sister came to Milan several times, demonstrating willingness to support the couple.

After two attempts and a risky pregnancy, Luisa was born. Now the couple sends me pictures of the little girl playing, eating, and sleeping. With a dedication each time, the same: "to the aunt in Milan."

16.33 Sophie and Aldo

Sophie is a Belgian woman (30 years old) in Italy for 5 years because of her marriage to Aldo, an entrepreneur, 51 years old. They present themselves at a PMA Center claiming that the prudent husband, at age 30, had proceeded with the cryopreservation of the semen. However, they appear disoriented and aimed at having a child at all costs, because of the age difference.

16.34 Sophie

Sophie lost her father at the age of 18 and stayed with her mother in the family home until her marriage. She sold the family business shortly before her wedding to provide her mother with a secure inheritance. She studied Finance in London and today in Italy manages large estates. She describes Aldo as "a miracle" a good, generous, paternal, emotionally fragile man, strong in life and in his profession. She fears being "alone" in the future, should her mother and husband pass away. A child would be a "good life insurance" and a "motivation beyond pain."

When I ask what the phrase "Aldo is a miracle" means, Sophie bursts into tears and describes the loss of her father as an ever-open wound. Her mother, after a few years, leaned on a friend of her husband, a family confidant, Christian, more for loneliness than for real necessity.

This man came to live with them 3 years after the loss of her husband. The first year, Sophie says, he was caring, he asked about my studies, he often came to visit me in London with my mother.

He insisted that I call him "dad" but I never managed to. This fact made him increasingly harsh in his relationship with me: he criticized my lifestyle, my friendships, my relationship "too close with my mother." Until one day during an argument over a trivial matter, he hit me and my mother who had run to mediate the situation.

We reported him but they were difficult years between lawyers, courts, and a life always in fear. My mother and I remained alone: our house became a bunker with alarm systems and a private night security service.

When I met Aldo, I did not fall in love easily. He waited without complaining, he helped my mother to resume social and recreational activities, he even suggested that she live with us in Italy. "My mother is Belgian to the core, she would never do it, but we see her often…".

16.35 Aldo

He married late because he did not believe in family and marriage. Above all, he did not think he could be a good husband and father. His family consisted of his parents and three brothers, before him, children from his father's first marriage, he was widowed after a car accident. Being a second marriage child, he was taught not to be a nuisance, not to cause problems, to be an "invisible" child. His brothers were much older: 15–10–8 years difference. With the third-born, he went to the park, to the zoo but "he called me DWARF." "I saw my mother was happy and that was enough for me. At 18 he left home: he attended evening Civil Engineering University and at 30 he started his own business." Speaking with a former university mate, he confided that he had undergone a spermogram and had been diagnosed as infertile. The confession significantly affected Aldo's sensitivity and thinking, and he proceeded to cryopreservation along with his study friend.

Marriage and a child had been put off for a long time, but having met Sophie he realized that with her he could create "a family within the family."

16.36 The Team

The team meeting was very intense and the specialists argued convincingly that the physical conditions of Sophie and Aldo offered much chance of success, even though Sophie's idiopathic infertility (and the lack of a sexuality appropriate to her young age) remained unclear.

It was decided to propose to the couple a couple of preparatory psychosexual meetings due to my perplexity about the real reasons for the desire for parenthood.

16.37 The Couple

During the interviews, the couple reflected a lot on their individual history, their relationship, and the hypoactive desire that had always conditioned the relationship. Unbeknownst to the entire team, however, the spouses turned to another fertility center, where they were immediately introduced into the PMA protocol.

Aldo called me on the phone revealing this step and apologizing for the decision. Sophie—he reported—had done everything by herself.

After about a year, Sophie and Aldo asked for a meeting. They appeared desperate and nullified. A PMA attempt and a miscarriage was the result of their experience. They are now in couple therapy to overcome the fear of death, the fear of being alone, and they are rebuilding a second couple contract.

16.38 Stefano and Lucrezia

They appear to be a very close couple with a strong emotional bond. They turn to a fertility center after failing a path of adoption that lasted 3 years. Now they want to try with a medical procreative procedure and set the limit to the team that they will undergo only one attempt. Stefano and Lucrezia work in the same Oil Company, but in different departments: "marketing" for him, "research" for her. They are respectively 43 years old (Stefano) and 39 years old (Lucrezia). They are both natives of Southern Italy: they both only have a mother and are the only children.

16.39 Stefano

With his smile, he immediately wins over the entire team. He tries to disguise the suffering experienced during the 3 years of the process for adoption. He reveals that psychologists and social workers have only done their job and that Lucrezia is the person, among the two, most emotionally tested. "Perhaps because she is the survivor of a twin birth," he suggests and is always ready to work for two, live for two, love for two. "The deceased sister is her recurring sense of guilt."

Later, Stefano says that his father was an alcoholic, the owner of a very successful wine shop. The mother, a secretary, managed the house and Stefano's education. "It's a pity that often my mother and I went to look for my father late at night and we would find him in a terrible state." My mother always defended me: "she had the strength to separate and to have sole custody. I always saw my father, my mother always respected him and only now do I understand the value of that behavior." Stefano declares himself a teetotaler and that he indulges wife and mother in all their desires. He is humiliated by the fact that sexually he suffers from secondary premature ejaculation (since he met Lucrezia) and wants a child "because he feels he can be a good father. Something he never had."

16.40 Lucrezia

They have been married for 7 years: they met during an organized trip to South Africa. They started the relationship immediately and after a year they got married. Lucrezia has a petite physique and suffers from primary anorgasmia. She reports that the adoption process was humiliating, demeaning, and devoid of humanity. "Every statement of mine was refuted, even the death of my father from a heart attack, while he was telling me about an employee of the firm (accountant). They made me feel inadequate, still mourning my father and emotionally more ready to take care of a handicapped child, than a newborn as per my wish." The mother remarried after 3 years and the relationship with the new partner was within the limits of education and respect. The Adoption Commission did not consider them suitable because "neither could bridge the gap between reason and gut feeling."

16.41 The Team

Certainly, the couple's history and the double presence of sexual dysfunctions made the geneticists' approach very cautious. In the meantime, they started the process for assisted medical procreation not without many difficulties. Many complications and poor compliance from the couple, more experienced in controlling than in being guided. The team agreed on the communicative style, it was agreed not to respond in the face of critical or judgmental attitudes of one or the other. It was agreed to lower as much as possible the expectations of success, not referring to statistics but to the fact "that they did not want to add more suffering to the couple" even in the orthodoxy of the medical procreative procedure. "By a miracle" as a geneticist said, Lucrezia became pregnant. "Also thanks to the sexological exercises that we did with great care and with which we finally experienced a real sexuality…," specifies Stefano.

16.42 Stefano and Lucrezia

The happiness of the achieved pregnancy was immediately conditioned by Lucrezia's fear of losing the baby. She resigned from work due to the pregnancy being at risk and from that moment she dedicated herself only to the good outcome of the pregnancy. She enrolled in "tai chi" and breathing courses in addition to the pre-birth course. Alessandro was born by cesarean section and the grandmothers were the most satisfied and happy people. Lucrezia went into postpartum depression, she refused to breastfeed the little one, and after a few months, panic attacks appeared. Stefano and Lucrezia are still followed psychologically because they feel unprepared to live as good parents. Even the grandmothers occasionally participate in therapy. Today Alessandro is 3 years old. He appears a smiling child, full of life and curious, albeit with some sleep disorder at night. Lucrezia and Stefano have decided to be 70% parents and 30% couple. They hired a "night nanny" full-time to feel more active during the day and closer to each other.

16.43 Giovanna and Giorgio

Giovanna presents herself alone at the umpteenth Infertility Center to undergo the fourth attempt at assisted reproduction. She justifies her husband's absence because they live in two different cities for professional reasons: Verona and Berlin.

16.44 Giovanna

The previous failures have increased Giovanna's anger and she does not intend to abandon any possible attempt. She complains about the lack of humanity of the previous specialists and declares a personal understanding on the subject of infertility through the internet and forums of women in her condition that have given her solidarity and comfort. The couple has been married for 5 years. They have known each other forever because the families of origin had socialized with each other since their adolescence. The long-distance relationship had fueled the desire for a child not a little.

Giorgio is 39 years old and Giovanna is 35. He works for an Italian textile company based in Germany. She owns a dog grooming shop.

Giorgio's absence appears very strange. The basic reason, explains Giovanna, is that she intercepted an SMS from her husband (who had returned home for the weekend) to his dearest friend. The message lamented Giovanna's perseverance in undergoing continuous IVF treatments, which the husband perceived as excessive stubbornness and lack of reasonableness. Although the friend urged him to stand by his wife and understand her deepest feelings, Giorgio replied that he was tired of the situation and that Giovanna was not taking care of him.

Giovanna experienced this message as abandonment.

16.45 Giorgio

An attempt was made to summon Giorgio to a meeting to give us further information and Giovanna did not want to be present. The husband expressed a clear intention to explore other options: adoption, fostering, volunteering, or accepting not to have children.

He appeared drained, exhausted by the long medical journey and terrified by another attempt at IVF. Giovanna had risked her life twice in previous attempts due to complications. The team decided to ask both for a meeting to assess the real chances of success of a fourth IVF attempt. Not many. Giovanna remained firm in her purpose and only when faced with the possibility of proceeding with a heterologous proposal from her husband, was she more conciliatory. They asked for a few days to reconsider. Another meeting was held: Giovanna in person, Giorgio on a video call from Berlin. The idea that a stranger would help them in their endeavor brought agreement: it could not be done. The child had to be natural and only theirs. They asked us for more time to reflect.

16.46 The Team and the Couple

After 2 years they presented themselves again for a couple's care. They had tried fostering with a not very edifying experience. For 3 months they had looked after a 13-year-old teenage girl who lived in a Community. The lack of experience of both made the girl start demanding trips, gifts, restaurant meals, and a choice of TV series to watch. In the end they gave in. "We made the mistake of bringing her to our house for a few hours," explained Giorgio "and it was the end. We realized that she was keeping tabs on us and using us as a benefit counter." "To our no," continued Giovanna, "she would throw herself on the ground, make hysterical scenes and once called the educator of the reference Community, telling him that we had beaten her." They appeared disoriented and victims of every possible sense of guilt for their inadequacy. They even questioned the reason why they got married and whether perhaps the search for a child was a palliative compared to their lack of emancipation. After a year of couple therapy, they mutually decided to separate.

16.47 Gregorio and Sara

Sara and Gregorio want a child and for 3 years they have investigated every type of cause to understand the lack of a pregnancy. They appear shocked by the diagnosis referred to them by more than one Fertility Center: "idiopathic infertility." They report having gone for consultation in the United States and the Netherlands, but nothing has changed. This time they appear irritated and no longer willing to do anything to become parents.

No one advises them to have a conversation with a psychosexual therapist to regain confidence in themselves.

16.48 Sara

A friend of Sara confides to her that she herself had turned to a psychologist for having risked severe depression during an IVF. With some reluctance, Sara decides to have a first interview. She appears distrustful and already inclined to assume that it is all a waste of time. She reports that she has been married for 5 years and has three older sisters (all married with children). She is 39 years old, works as a criminal lawyer in her husband's office, a civil lawyer, 41 years old, and the only child, with a Somali mother and Italian father. During the interview, she feels very frustrated because her mother-in-law cannot conceive of a marriage without children "also because if she hadn't had any, left by her husband, she would never have come to Italy with Gregorio" because she would have become a "disowned wife."

16.49 Gregorio

He presents himself at the second interview with Sara and reports that he studied in Italy from the age of 7 and that he feels more Italian than Italian-Somali. His mother Chewi is very rooted in Somali culture and above all, she feels very lonely. She lives in a neighborhood away from the couple, is reserved, and attends the Somali community once a week. They appear to be a couple very committed professionally, with little time for hobbies and friends. Gregorio is very attached to Sara's family of origin and tends to downplay his mother's false beliefs. Their trips to the United States and Holland are motivated by "we were already there for work, we combined business with pleasure…." He is very worried about the fact that Sara's great-grandmother was always a depressed person, with multiple admissions to Psychiatric Departments first and in Psychiatric Communities to follow, until suicide at the age of 55. He thinks that such a family history can be transmissible and, in that case, the newborn could suffer from this pathology. He confesses this fear in the therapeutic context and Sara, taken aback, "why didn't you talk to me about it? Doctor, believe me, I didn't know anything…".

16.50 The Couple and the Team

The team informed of these assumptions, it is decided to have Sara undergo ovulation stimulation. Gregorio appears increasingly anxious. They come to interviews with me until Sara becomes pregnant with twins. After the birth, fears follow that the babies may not be healthy and both parents hypothesize: autism, rare diseases, emotional disorders.

For the entire first year of life, they met me to have reassurances, vent their anxieties, talk about the progress of the children. They refused Gregorio's mother's advice to show the children to a Somali doctor. After weaning the children, they realized that the fears had gradually dissipated. Today they have three children: 2 years after the birth of the twins, Jacopo was born.

16.51 Conclusions

Although medical scientific research shows that only 5% of infertile couples experience dysfunctional sexuality, these life stories are exhaustive of how many relational, affective, sexual elements converge in the history of a couple. Both the children born and the little ones never born remain in the hearts of couples making them in both cases "parents": just for the fact of having invested so much and having loved them from the beginning, even more than themselves. Family histories, not always resolved, condition not a little the projects of a couple who often do not have the time to build their own "culture of life as a couple."

Explaining all this would be very useful to geneticists, urologists–andrologists, endocrinologists, gynecologists, who are still trained in biological causes and not in people. Often couples ignore the fact that even if they are the cause of problems, they can also be the only solution to their problem. There is still much to do in this regard and it is the task of the most organized teams to educate colleagues and couples not to be afraid to ask for a psychosexual consultation, when it is not offered.

In my professional years, I have collected photos of children and couples who want to testify with an image, their dreams, desires, and difficulties.

A heritage for me and my colleagues that always reminds us to live with an inch of humility above fear.

16.52 Letter from a Father to a Son

I watch you in the evening as you fall asleep and I feel happy, full of life. I hope that you sleep and that you will not wake me up in a few hours with screams and shouts… you know I discovered that if I put on the Beatles tape and we dance together you fall asleep immediately. Mom says that I spoil you but you know that your dad as a child only slept if my father sang to me "how cold your little hand is..let me warm it…" Better the Beatles than the opera: we are pop.

Then, when you say to your friend "watch it, I'm going to tell my dad" I will feel triumphant and the best of dads, your bodyguard.

Mom says that I have to prepare for my sunset as a hero. When you tell me "Pietro's dad has a motorcycle, why don't you ride a motorcycle? " Sure, other dads will be the best heroes from then on but I will make up for it when, scolded by mom, you tell her "tonight I'm going to tell my dad."

I already imagine you with me at our team's game at the stadium or older, having a beer "just us men" or telling each other that mom is nagging…but woe if she wasn't there…

Now I look at you and I feel alive. I look at you and I am moved thinking about you little one, that I never had…

Chapter 17
Vademecum for the Couple

Clinical experience has shown a series of psychological and relational references that couples often disregard because in all of them the desire for a child prevails and nothing else:

1. When approaching a medical methodology for infertility, every couple should hypothesize more outcomes: becoming parents, remaining in the relationship as a couple, adoption or foster care, volunteering in pediatric clinical or recreational facilities.
2. Having more projects produces greater cohesion in the couple, avoids pursuing false dreams, eliminates the risk of a medical insistence without congruent outcomes.
3. The couple, no matter how disoriented, emotionally tested, conditioned by the feeling that infertility has transformed them into a second-rate couple, must present themselves to the centers for infertility treatment, as "protagonists of their own projectuality."
4. Clinicians, in perfect good faith, will see them as individuals in difficulty, but it is up to the couple to remember that they have all the tools to face the Clinical process and they are not just "patients." They are people in their entirety.
5. Alongside visits and laboratory tests, asking for psychosexual consultations is a way to experience clinicians in a relationship "on equal terms." They will dedicate themselves to genetics, the couple to their own motivation, to foresee or go through moments of stress, anxiety, and misunderstanding.
6. When starting a clinical journey, many couples live unexpressed fears and anxieties of failure. Confronting with a psychosexual therapist avoids marginalization, loneliness, discouragement. This figure will act as a liaison with the rest of the team to share a communicative modality suitable for the couple, an individualized approach.

E. V. Longhi, *Framing Sexual Dysfunctions and Diseases during Fertility Treatment*, https://doi.org/10.1007/978-3-031-76726-5_17

7. If the partners appear to be the people who express the most anxiety and depression, the partners are not exempt from feelings of guilt, a sense of inadequacy, and of inability to make the partner happy.
8. Many couples protect each other by avoiding talking about their own fragilities: it is necessary to remember that the relationship is on equal terms, it is not a parental relationship between mother–son and father–daughter.
9. Personal histories and the couple's history are the essential conditions to make clinicians understand: at what point in the life of the couple the desire for a child was nurtured, how many children there should be (of the families of origin, of social prejudices or to even the score with friends who have already become parents, and so on), the meaning of the birth of a child in relation to personal history (sister/brother with children, previous abortions, divorces caused by the absence of children in previous unions, preexisting diseases).
10. The history of the couple's sexuality is another necessary element to know in what way sexuality is confused or connected with fertility in the couple's history. Previous experiences with dysfunctional or frigid partners intensifies the desire for a child to definitively eliminate the problem of intimacy.
11. The families of origin, whether complicit or dissenting, in this journey can be a severe conditioning in the clinical and psychological compliance of the couple. The psychosexual therapist can help support the couple in times of great family tension, setting boundaries between the individual role of children and the adult role of the couple. Many individuals appear "forever" dependent on parental judgment. But what will become of that child? Who will they have as parents: the grandparents or the couple? Worse, how many parents will they have to face?
12. Miscarriages represent a moment of great crisis and pain between the couple members. Often this discomfort is shared "in time" with friends or relatives, but the couple will "always" live this event, questioning the physical health of their own bodies, as well as their mental integrity.
13. Asking for a Psychosexual Specialist, when they are not already part of the clinical team process, is not a declaration of incapacity. It is an act of courage. It means that the most fragile part of our feelings needs to be constantly nourished, in different times and ways. Not in solitude. And especially with someone who, knowing the impact of fertility procedures, prepares the couple for possible future scenarios.
14. Medical language is often incomprehensible and very technical. Meeting a "facilitator," who translates medical language into more everyday terminology, can improve the couple's harmony and synergy with the medical team.
15. Logic leads to thinking "I must do it alone" and "we must do it alone" because it is easier to accept a disease on which a clinician can help us, rather than facing an unknown scenario, admitting to "not having calculated the right emotional price together."
16. Just as marathon runners feel a moment of "crisis" during the most ambitious and exhausting races, every couple has a clinical time to react to therapies, an emotional and relational time to deal with reality. Presupposing a priori during the journey that there will inevitably be moments of relational "fatigue" or

"adjustment crisis" is one of the ways to overcome in team what in couple would lead to apathy, fights, suffering, or abandonment of therapies.

17. Every couple should also measure themselves with the idea "when to say enough." Often infertility therapies "depersonalize," we feel like machines that "work or are broken." Setting a limit in advance is a way to respect oneself, avoiding overestimating physical, emotional, and sexual abilities.
18. Sexuality during procreative paths results in "a calendar," loses spontaneity, naturalness, and the sexual dysfunctions of one or both partners are experienced as a limit compared to the child-goal. In reality, it is a way in which the couple says: "there is no time and space for us."
19. Even when the outcome of therapies is successful, pregnancy, childbirth, breast-feeding, weaning, and so on are extremely tiring stages for parents intensely tried for a long or medium time, and who must return to the usual work and social burdens.
20. Couples living in different contexts from their places of origin find themselves dealing with another type of "loneliness" compared to that of infertility. This causes tensions both within the couple and in intra- and extra-family relationships. And sexuality waits…often to disappear for a long time.
21. Often couples become accomplices "only to solve problems": the growth of the newborn, the difficulties of breastfeeding, daily management, economic administration, the division of tasks, the depression of a new mother with much fear of not being up to it.
22. You become parents before generating a child. It is necessary to reflect that you cannot be parents if you are not an adult couple. Setting boundaries between these roles is not always consequent: talking to a psychosexologist, who perhaps has followed you since the first access to the Infertility Clinic, is a way to acquire awareness with your own two goals and your own individual judgments of authoritative scarcity.
23. Cultural, social, religious, economic, and geographical belonging are living conditions that differentiate couples in various contexts and in various states. It is important to know the culture of origin of the couples because they attribute different values and meanings of the conjugal, parental, filial, friendly, professional, and gender relationship.
24. Building together with couples and for couples "single therapeutic teams" is certainly an optimal goal: for the couples and for the team.
25. The psychosexologist is not for life: but is a facilitator for a time, for the necessary time for every type of couple and team.
26. The perception of infertility implies an experience to share and face. It also involves living infertility as a common project, acquiring understanding and comfort, sharing emotions and crying together. Processing infertility together with the spouse involves revealing thoughts on infertility, describing sensations openly, using humor in difficult situations, and promoting a spirit of union.
27. The "combative" attitude implies perseverance, the ability to recover and gather strength after disappointment, trying to control the situation and focusing on the moment. Accepting the negative emotions promotes coping and includes giving

in to all types of emotions such as pain, anger, and rage, in addition to experiencing a series of other emotions. Moreover, expressing feelings of fear and despair through "writing" promotes coping.

28. Emotional control involves the conscious exclusion of self-contempt, pain, negative feelings, and anger, as well as putting an end to the avoidance of families with children.
29. Maintaining a good condition, taking care of one's well-being, having good self-esteem, and selecting thoughts (choosing only those "neutral or positive" on which one can build individually and as a couple) are the most fruitful premises for planning as many futures as possible.
30. The decision-making process regarding infertility treatments also includes taking a break from the treatments themselves to regain emotional and physical strength as well as considering further alternatives.
31. "Reprogramming the future" implies seeing other goals beyond parenthood, making alternative plans for the future, and trying to enjoy all aspects of life. Making major changes to one's existence promotes old dormant desires such as resuming abandoned studies, planning the search for a new job, selecting acquaintances, and favoring loyal friends. Moreover, in some cases, it also leads to divorce and/or the adoption of a child.

Chapter 18
Sexual Dysfunction in Postpartum Women

Pregnancy is generally a particularly delicate time to address sexual health problems [1]. Especially for infertile women who have undergone a long diagnostic, therapeutic journey among fears of failure and unsuccessful attempts. The World Health Organization (WHO) has suggested that it is necessary to conduct research on sexual health and has consistently emphasized the need to provide assistance, information, and prenatal and postpartum counseling to women [2].

The criteria of the Diagnostic and Statistical Manual of Mental Disorders, fifth edition (DSM-5) for female sexual dysfunction state that sexual symptoms are present for a minimum duration of about 6 months, causing clinically significant discomfort in the woman and her partner [3]. We can therefore hypothesize that for an infertile patient the times are longer and a source of anxiety, depression, anhedonia. This is compounded by the fact that there is not enough dialogue between women and health workers on female sexual health [4]. Women do not discuss their concerns with doctors, and specialists often exclude a priori screening on sexual health [5]. They themselves (the doctors) do not have confidence in addressing sexual health problems and often underestimate the prevalence of female sexual dysfunctions and the negative physical, psychological, and emotional consequences [6].

Even the sexual function of fertile women decreases during pregnancy and remains low during the postpartum period [7]. The literature has shown that there is an association between pregnancy and sexual dysfunction [8]:

1. In the first trimester of pregnancy, sexual desire often decreases due to exhaustion, nausea, emotional lability, and increased anxiety or fear of a miscarriage. In the second trimester, there is an increase in libido as physical symptoms decrease, vaginal lubrication improves and previous anxiety decreases as women psychologically adapt to pregnancy.
2. In the third trimester, the physical difficulties that women usually experience make sexual activities more uncomfortable and less frequent. Studies on female sexual function during pregnancy have shown that during the first trimester, 96%

E. V. Longhi, *Framing Sexual Dysfunctions and Diseases during Fertility Treatment*, https://doi.org/10.1007/978-3-031-76726-5_18

of pregnant women had vaginal intercourse, but in the third trimester only 67% continued to have intimate relationships.
3. In the first, second, and third trimester of pregnancy, respectively, 66.3%, 50.7% and 69.2% of women experienced sexual dysfunctions, with sexual desire disorder appearing as the most often reported sexual dysfunction in each trimester [9].
4. Studies have found that during pregnancy, only 11.2% of pregnant women showed favorable attitudes toward sexuality [10]. Furthermore, 68% of the women interviewed admitted that they had never talked about sexual problems with their doctor while they were pregnant.

Infertile women often confuse the concepts of sexuality and fertility, so, in the case of a much-desired pregnancy, they omit any kind of intimacy to "not lose the baby" or "not harm it." As a result, after childbirth, they see themselves only as mothers and no longer as partners.

This is also because for a long time they have experienced feelings of low self-esteem, emotional discomfort, anxiety, and symptoms of depression [11]. Not only: the female sexual function becomes increasingly dysfunctional due to the stress related to labor and childbirth, the lack of support from the partner, the increase in responsibility associated with having a child, and the lack of independence [12].

On the other hand, the partner feels, following the emotional and physical burn out during infertility treatments, to be able to "catch their breath and think about themselves" by immersing themselves in work. The lack of sexual activity in couples continues during breastfeeding and the weaning of the little one, encouraging conflicts, mood alteration, and marital dissatisfaction. Everything is centered on the newborn: even the discussions between the new parents. Anxieties are fueled by the lack of the little one's night sleep or the difficulty of the newborn to attach to the mother's breast. "In the first three months of my son's life" a new father reported "we went to the pediatric emergency room at least ten times. And always at night: for overfeeding or gassy colic or for the baby's constant awakenings. In the end we looked for a 'sleep nanny' …" The increase in household expenses often justifies fathers to stay late in the evening or to incentivize overtime, especially if the grandparents live in other regions and the couple does not benefit from help in the daily management of the little one.

This is why couples should already ask during the period of fertility treatments and prenatal care for a psychosexual consultation. The sexual anamnesis of the couple and an evaluation of the partner pre-, during, and post pregnancy could help couples to remain such, even with the birth of a child and, to improve the quality of the relationship. The most burdensome transition for infertile couples (in particular) is indeed separating the role of the adult couple from the parental couple.

The link between postpartum depression and sexual dysfunctions has been well studied. Depression can cause a decrease in sexual desire, reducing interest in sexual activity. Pregnancy often brings changes in lower physical, emotional, and neurological resistance. Depression can amplify the feeling of tiredness, making it difficult to engage in sexual activity and influencing the sexual response. Depression can also put a strain on relationships and lead to emotional distance or communication difficulties between partners. This tension can create barriers in intimacy and in the less empathetic and more symmetric relationship between partners [13].

As suggested by the study of Ozerdogan et al. [14], the development of FSD during pregnancy continues inexorably in the postpartum period. Addressing sexual dysfunction during pregnancy can help prevent a painful and inadequate sexual response postpartum and promote postpartum recovery.

Sexual dysfunction is a common problem in women in the last trimester of pregnancy and the 8 weeks after childbirth. However, whereas this problem is substantially resolved after 6 months from childbirth, infertile women risk worsening and, in the best-case scenario, prolonging over time. A surprising discovery emerged in this study is the increase in the risk of depression in the sixth month after childbirth when women generally start working.

But there is more.

The study by Yurt and Çankaya [15] determined the effects of post-traumatic stress disorder (PTSD) on maternal adaptation and infant perception in primiparous mothers after childbirth. A total of 378 mothers who had given birth 6–8 weeks earlier were recruited. Of the 378 mothers who participated in the study, 97 (25.7%) scored above the threshold value of the post-traumatic stress scale (≥33). After vaginal delivery, it was found that primiparous mothers with post-traumatic stress disorder in the postpartum period had a more disturbed maternal adaptation and infant perception. It was also established that primiparous mothers with post-traumatic stress disorder who had experienced a traumatic birth reported difficulty adapting to motherhood and showed problems in perception, acceptance, and bonding with the newborn.

If this situation concerns only fertile women, we can hypothesize that scientific research should investigate the post-traumatic stress of infertile patients, whose mental state is already very disturbed in the search for reproductive therapies. If perineal traumas during childbirth, primiparity at an advanced age, increased depression, anxiety, relationship dissatisfaction in the postpartum period were added, the risk of permanent sexual dysfunctions would reach a very high level. The data were collected using a multidimensional questionnaire, such as the Female Sexual Function Index, the Depression Anxiety and Stress Scale, and the Relationship Assessment Scale. Sixty-six percent of patients scored below the limit value (<26.5) for sexual dysfunction [14].

On the other hand, it seems that sexual dysfunction was less in multiparous women compared to primiparous women ($p = 0.006$). A low sexual activity in primiparous women can be due to less privacy and a greater loss of time and energy. Several factors, including the living situation, monthly income, the incision of the episiotomy, and the couple's level of education, were influential on the sexual function of primiparous women ($p < 0.05$). Sexual function differs between primiparous and multiparous women in the postpartum period and the number of births can affect sexual performance [16].

Lacking further studies on the subject, the fact remains that severe perineal injuries are associated with persistent dyspareunia ($p < 0.05$). Postpartum dyspareunia is independently influenced by operative delivery, previous dyspareunia, recurrent urogenital infections, and urgency incontinence The fact remains that it significantly compromises the sexual health of women after childbirth, mainly caused by perineal traumas due to childbirth management and recurrent urogenital infections [17].

Studies suggest that a third to half of fertile patients have experienced childbirth as positive [18] and a fifth have reported having experienced childbirth as negative or traumatic [19]. Negative birth experiences are particularly important because of their potential impact on women and their families. Most of the research in this area has attempted to understand negative and traumatic birth experiences, focusing on their nature, evaluation, risk factors, and protective factors. A review of the predictors and outcomes of the childbirth experience has identified a lack of literature regarding positive birth experiences, or even neutral, with greater attention to the identification of risk factors for post-traumatic stress disorder (or stress symptoms) following childbirth.

For infertile couples, the situation is far more complex. Patients arrive at childbirth in a psychological condition at the limit and their partners share the anguish due to the possible risk of life of the woman during childbirth, complications, or the risk of a malformed or frail newborn. It is no coincidence that often the couple falls into an anhedonic state that deprives them of sexual desire. Post-traumatic stress postpartum manifests the fatigue of the central nervous system and the emotional resilience of the couple from the beginning of fertility treatments, through the number of attempts, pregnancy, and childbirth. A stressful journey that finds the new parents without emotional reserves. The sight of the long-desired baby often ambivalently induces joy and insensitivity toward the newborn. Breastfeeding, care, weaning, variability of sleep hours, the tight spaces for the couple, the lack of freedom, and so on influence in no small way the hypoactive desire, almost as if to say that after so much effort "there is no room for intimacy for two. We need to wait for a moment when the couple will be freer" When?

18.1 Conclusions

The absence of a clear vision of the clinical and emotional processes that the couple will have to face deprives them of a projection on the possible scenarios that could alternate over time in the long or medium term. Specialists and sexologists should work in this sense. The infertile couple only has in mind to become parents at all costs and the idea is not yet widespread that they should be guided in the investment of emotional resources, in going through crisis moments, in foreseeing disappointment, fatigue, and loneliness. The emotional distance, often of doctors who still ask "do you want to talk to a psychologist?" (and do not admit that having information from the start about the stability of the couple can be an important condition of their compliance in the fertilization process), makes individuals feel perpetually inadequate patients. "Like the psychologist? We are not mentally ill" is the prejudice of many couples who live their infertility as a social stigma. Showing infertile couples that the medical team needs further information (psychological, sexual, on the social network of the couple) would offer individuals a "certainty of accompaniment and investment in each of them" One infertile couple asked me "but how many are you who follow us? We have never had so many people for us. Are we a difficult case?" Having more reference figures is neither disorienting nor dispersive, as long as the team shows cohesion, esteem, respect, and above all, great trust in the resources of the couple, regardless of the final outcome.

References

1. DeJudicibus MA, McCabe MP (2002) Psychological factors and sexuality of women during pregnancy and after childbirth. J Sex Res 39:94–103. https://doi.org/10.1080/00224490209552128
2. World Health Organization (2006) Definition of sexual health: report of a technical consultation on sexual health, 28–31 January 2002. World Health Organization, Geneva, pp 1–35
3. The criteria of the Diagnostic and Statistical Manual of Mental Disorders, 5th edition (DSM-5) for female sexual dysfunction require that sexual symptoms be present for a minimum duration of about 6 months, causing clinically significant discomfort in the individual.
4. Politi MC, Clark MA, Armstrong G, McGarry KA, Sciamanna CN (2009) Patient-provider communication on sexual health among unmarried middle-aged and older women. J Gen Intern Med 24:511–516. https://doi.org/10.1007/s11606-009-0930-z
5. Kingsberg SA (2006) Collection of a sexual history. Obstet Gynecol Clin N Am 33:535–547. https://doi.org/10.1016/j.ogc.2006.09.002
6. Peck SA (2001) The importance of sexual health history in the context of primary care. J Obstet Gynecol Neonatal Nurses 30:269–274. https://doi.org/10.1111/j.1552-6909.2001.tb01544.x
7. O'Malley D, Higgins A, Begley C, Daly D, Smith V (2018) Prevalence and risk factors associated with sexual health problems in primiparous women at 6 and 12 months postpartum; a prospective longitudinal cohort study (the MAMMI study). BMC Pregnancy Childbirth 18:196. https://doi.org/10.1186/s12884-018-1838-6
8. Bartellas E, Crane JM, Daley M, Bennett KA, Hutchens D (2000) Sexuality and sexual activity in pregnancy. BJOG 107:964–968. https://doi.org/10.1111/j.1471-0528.2000.tb10397.x
9. Bayrami R, Sattarzadeh N, Koochaksariie FR, Pezeshki MZ (2008) Sexual dysfunction in couples and related factors during pregnancy. J Reprod Infertil 9:271–282
10. Khalesi ZB, Simbar M, Azin SA, Zayeri F (2016) Interventions and strategies for promoting public sexual health: a qualitative study. Electron Physician 8:2489–2496. https://doi.org/10.19082/2489
11. Nik-Azin A, Nainian MR, Zamani M, Bavojdan MR, Bavojdan MR, Motlagh MJ (2013) Evaluation of sexual function, quality of life, and mental and physical health in pregnant women. J Family Reprod Health 7:171–176
12. Witting K, Santtila P, Alanko K, Harlaar N, Jern P, Johansson A, Von Der Pahlen B, Varjonen M, Algars M, Sandnabba NK (2008) Female sexual function and its associations with number of children, pregnancy, and relationship satisfaction. J Sex Marital Ther 34:89–106. https://doi.org/10.1080/00926230701636163
13. McCool-Myers M, Theurich M, Zuelke A, Knuettel H, Apfelbacher C (2018) Predictors of female sexual dysfunction: a systematic review and qualitative analysis through gender inequality paradigms. BMC Womens Health 18:108. https://doi.org/10.1186/s12905-018-0602-4
14. Ozerdogan N, Mizrak SB, Gursoy E, Zeren F (2022) Sexual dysfunction in the third trimester of pregnancy and postpartum period: a prospective longitudinal study. J Obstet Gynecol 42:2722–2728. https://doi.org/10.1080/01443615.2022.2106830

15. Yurt G, Çankaya S (2023) Effects of post-traumatic stress disorder on maternal adaptation and perception of the newborn in the postpartum period. Early Child Dev Care 193(3):388–400. https://doi.org/10.1080/03004430.2022.2093867
16. Banaei M, Alidost F, Ghasemi E, Dashti S (2020) A comparison between sexual function in primiparous and multiparous women. J Obstet Gynecol 40(3):411–418. https://doi.org/10.1080/01443615.2019.1640191
17. Bertozzi S, Londero AP, Fruscalzo A, Driul L, Marchesoni D (2010) Prevalence and risk factors for dyspareunia and unsatisfactory sexual relations in a cohort of first-time and second-time mothers 12 months after childbirth. Int J Sex Health 22(1):47–53. https://doi.org/10.1080/19317610903408130
18. Michels A, Kruske S, Thompson R (2013) Women's postnatal psychological functioning: the role of satisfaction with intrapartum care and the birth experience. J Reprod Infant Psychol 31(2):172–182. https://doi.org/10.1080/02646838.2013.791921
19. Simpson M, Catling C (2016) Understanding the experiences of psychological traumatic births: a review of the literature. Women Birth 29(3):203–207. https://doi.org/10.1016/j.wombi.2015.10.009

Chapter 19
Artificial Intelligence and Infertility

Studies on the use of artificial intelligence could facilitate pregnancies in older women at the edge of their fertile age. In these stages, the incidence of embryos with chromosomal abnormalities (aneuploidy) results in serious clinical consequences such as infertility, spontaneous abortion, and birth defects [1].

Experts in the field of reproductive medicine have invested their efforts in the selection and transfer of the single most vital embryo that will lead to the birth of a healthy child. The reduction in the number of embryos transferred confers numerous advantages to the patient, including the reduction of overall health costs, the minimization of potential complications, and the reduction of the mental, physical, and emotional burden resulting from repeated implantation failures and pregnancy losses [2].

This selection process presents itself as one of the main challenges in the field of in vitro fertilization (IVF). The evaluation of embryonic morphology by an expert embryologist on day 3 or day 5 of development has been the predominant noninvasive means to assess the quality of the embryo and the subsequent selection for transfer [3]. This technology allows embryologists to monitor the development of the embryo and to perform morphokinetic analyses with greater ease, leading to an improvement in implantation potential and pregnancy rate [4]. Although morphological evaluation and morphokinetic annotations are noninvasive, the two methods are time-consuming and may present the disadvantage of intra-observer and inter-observer variability, due to their inherent subjectivity [5].

STORK-A was designed to noninvasively predict embryonic ploidy. Using a dataset with images at 110 h after intracytoplasmic sperm injection and clinical information for 10,378 embryos, several machine learning and deep learning models were developed to assess which features contribute to the classification of ploidy. Maternal age, along with morphological evaluation, were strong predictors of embryonic ploidy, while morphokinetic parameters did not contribute to improving predictions.

E. V. Longhi, *Framing Sexual Dysfunctions and Diseases during Fertility Treatment*, https://doi.org/10.1007/978-3-031-76726-5_19

However, STORK-A is still an experimental study. It correctly predicts euploid embryos and single aneuploid embryos that could be used to supplement traditional methods of selection and prioritization of embryos.

Some studies have been published on PubMed and Google Scholar from January 1, 2000 to June 5, 2021 (using the search terms ["ivf" OR "in vitro fertilization"] AND "embryo selection" AND "quality" AND "ploidy" AND "aneuploid" AND "euploid" AND "artificial intelligence" OR "machine learning" OR "deep learning"). However, the path of research to predict the ploidy status of the embryo as a standardized method of embryo selection still seems long.

The challenge remains open for the evaluation of morphological quality and morphokinetic analysis. Even a third method, preimplantation genetic testing for aneuploidy (PGT-A), has its limitations, including invasiveness and costs. It is good for all clinicians and patients to know these ongoing processes without neglecting the complexity of the human being and their perception of life.

References

1. Herbert M, Kalleas D, Cooney D, Lamb M, Lister L (2015) Meiosis and maternal aging: insights from aneuploid oocytes and trisomy births. Cold Spring Harb Perspect Biol 7:a017970
2. Barnes J, Brendel M, Gao VR, Rajendran S, Kim J, Li Q, Malmsten JE, Sierra JT, Zisimopoulos P, Sigaras A, Khosravi P, Meseguer M, Zhan Q, Rosenwaks Z, Elemento O, Zaninovic N, Hajirasouliha I (2023) A non-invasive artificial intelligence approach for the prediction of human blastocyst ploidy: a retrospective model development and validation study. Lancet Digit Health 5(1):e28–e40. https://doi.org/10.1016/S2589-7500(22)00213-8
3. Gardner DK, Sakkas D (2003) Assessment of embryo vitality: the ability to select a single embryo for transfer: a review. Placenta 24(supplement B):S5–S12
4. Meseguer M, Rubio I, Cruz M, Basile N, Marcos J, Requena A (2012) Incubation and selection of the embryo in a time-lapse monitoring system improves pregnancy outcome compared to a standard incubator: a retrospective cohort study. Fertil Steril 98:1481–9.e10
5. Khosravi P, Kazemi E, Zhan Q et al (2019) Deep learning enables robust assessment and selection of human blastocysts after in vitro fertilization. NPJ Digit Med 2:21

The manufacturer's authorised representative in the EU is Springer Nature Customer Service Centre GmbH, Europaplatz 3, 69115 Heidelberg, Germany. If you have any concerns regarding our products, please contact ProductSafety@springernature.com

Printed and bound by CPI Group (UK) Ltd, Croydon, CR0 4YY

07/07/2026

02160911-0001